A Textbook of

Hospital and Clinical Pharmacy

(For Degree Course)

A Textbook of Hospital and Clinical Pharmacy

(For Degree Course)

Dr. Anees A. Siddiqui
Faculty of Pharmacy, Jamia Hamdard,
New Delhi - 110 062

Seemi Siddiqui
B.Pharm
SGC College of Pharmacy,
Ahera, Baghpat

Imran Parvez
B.Pharm., MBA
Regional Manager,
Ranbaxy Pvt. Ltd., Gurgaon

CBS

CBS PUBLISHERS & DISTRIBUTORS PVT. LTD.
New Delhi • Bengaluru • Chennai • Kochi • Mumbai • Pune

ISBN : 978-81-239-1672-9

First Edition : 2009
Reprint : 2011, 2014

Published by Satish Kumar Jain and produced by V.K. Jain for
CBS Publishers & Distributors Pvt. Ltd.,
CBS Plaza, 4819/XI Prahlad Street, 24 Ansari Road, Daryaganj,
New Delhi - 110002, India. • Website: www.cbspd.com
e-mail: delhi@cbspd.com, cbspubs@airtelmail.in
Ph.: 23289259, 23266861, 23266867 • Fax: 011-23243014

Branches:

- ***Bengaluru:*** Seema House, 2975, 17th Cross, K.R. Road, Bansankari 2nd Stage, Bengaluru - 560070
  • Ph.: +91-80-26771678/79 • Fax: +91-80-26771680
  • E-mail: cbsbng@gmail.com, bangalore@cbspd.com
- ***Pune:*** Bhuruk Prestige, Sr. No. 52/12/2+1+3/2, Narhe, Haveli (Near Katraj-Dehu Road By-pass), Pune - 411041
  • Ph.: +91-20-64704058/59, 32342277 • E-mail: pune@cbspd.com
- ***Kochi:*** 36/14, Kalluvilakam, Lissie Hospital Road, Kochi - 682018, Kerala • Ph.: +91-484-4059061-65
  • Fax: +91-484-4059065 • E-mail: cochin@cbspd.com
- ***Chennai:*** 20, West Park Road, Shenoy Nagar, Chennai - 600030
  Ph.: +91-44-26260666, 26208620 • Fax: +91-44-42032115
  • E-mail: chennai@cbspd.com

Printed at :
J.S. Offset Printers, Delhi

Preface

The subject, 'Hospital and Clinical Pharmacy', was not included in the pharmacy curriculum in India earlier whether it is diploma or degree course. The curriculum was designed to fulfil the need of pharmaceutical industry but during the last two decade, this subject has started its inception. Hence, this subject is introduced in the pharmacy curriculum and PG course related to clinical pharmacy field has also been started. Although, the subject 'Hospital and Clinical Pharmacy' has been introduced but it is difficult to find an appropriate book for the guidance.

The present book has been compiled to provide the elementary knowledge to this field and fulfil the need of students pursuing the pharmacy course. The book has been compiled to cover the topics of the syllabus prescribed in most of the universities in India.

The book is divided into three Sections, consisting of 25 Chapters. The Section I, II and III are related to Hospital Pharmacy, Clinical Pharmacy and Practical Exercises respectively. The main task of the book is to present the subjects in simple and understandable style for the benefit of the students.

The authors are thankful for continuing association and help of Shri S.K. Jain and Shri V.K. Jain, M/s CBS Publishers and Distributors for releasing this book. We are thankful to Mrs. Rafat Siddiqui for providing support for this book.

We have tried every effort to avoid typographic errors. However, despite best efforts, some might have appear in inadvertently. We shall be obliged if these are brought to our notice.

Date : July, 2008 **Authors**

1

Chapter

Hospital

A **hospital** is an institution for health care providing treatment by specialised staff and equipment, and often but not always providing for longer-term patient stays. The word 'hospital' is derived from the latin word hospitium which means a place where guests are receoved. A hospital is a complicated organization containing specilized testing laboratories, scientific eqipments and team of trained professsional people educated to the prolems concerning with heath and hygeine. All these are united together to restore and maimtain good health of the public.

History

The concept of foundation of hospitals was given by Arabs. The King Walid bin Abdal Malik founded the first hospital in 707 A.D. and appointed physician to work there. A hospital was started by Add-al-Dawlah in Baghdad in 997 A.D. with 24 physician. In Cairo, the largest hospital built in 1283. A mobile hospital was eastablihed in Baghdad in 942 A.D. which was seen to different parts where prisoners were lodged or where epidemic broke out. Some hospitals were founded during 12th and 13th century in Turkey. Some hospitals were founded by women with the spirit of charity. The Arabs establihed special eye hospitals and mental asylum. The well equipped hospitals offered every opportunity to students to learn about medicine in practical way. Records of interesting and useful observations were kept there. Elaborate studies were made of symptomatology of nervous and skin diseases, veneral diseases, epidermology, and opthalmology. The cataract operation by incision and dry suction, and many other operaions were undertaken and performed successively. Only those physician were allowed to practise medicine who passed a prescribed test.

Muhammad bin Tughlaq (1325-1351) built more than seventy hospital in India. His successor, Firoz Shah Tughlaq, added five more hospitals. These hospitals had competent physicians and well stocked with medicines and other provisions. Akbar, the Great built a large hospital at Fatehpur Sikri. The other mughal successors also built hospitals at Delhi, Ahmedabad, Surat, Etawah, etc. The Ayurvedic and Unani physicians worked in these hospitals.

The first allopathic hospitals were founded by Spanish in Mexico city in 1525 and French in Canada. The earlier hospitals had the lodging for the poor and needy. Mainly the pilgrims and wayfarers were admitted in them. Later on the laprosy patients were accommodated in these hospitals. The socially depressed, physically handicapped, financially weak and the sick persons were kept together. During small pox epidemics, hospital tok care of sick. Generally, they were run for the homeless sick. They were considered a last resort, since the death rate was very high.

Hospital Concept in India

The establishment of hospitals in India for treating patients according to modern (allopathic) system of medicine can be credited to the Dutch, the French, the Portuguese and the British (East India) trading companies and their military adventures. These hospitals initially were meant for their nationals and persons in their employment. The military establishment had their units exclusively meant for their use. The misssionaries set up clean and efficient charitable dispensories and hospitals for the public at large. The municiplities also set up new hospitals with the help of generous donors or with their own funds. The provicinal ruling authorities became interested and they set up medical colleges with attached hospitals. Other facilities were added by private donors, chartable foundations and service clubs (Rotatary, Lions, Masons, etc.). The Drugs Enquiry Committee report of 1931 (Chopra Committee) mentioned that there was neither profession of pharmacy nor facilities to train qualified pharmacists. The picture changed with the establishment of the first department in the country devoted in training in pharmaceutical subjects at Banaras. Since then many new insititutes/colleage/university have come into existence and several thousands of pharmacists trained but it is sad to record that hospital pharmacy has been neglected and this branch of the profession is still in its infancy in our country.

All over the world, qualified pharmacists practice their profession community pharmacist or as hospital pharmacists but unfortunately in India qualified pharmacists are mostly employed in the industry due to their better prospects. There are very few opportunities in India for qualified pharmacists in hospitals. The pay package and promotion chances are also unattractive, the perquisites are missing and the prestige associated with the post of a hospital pharmacist missing in the society. A hospital pharmacist in the deloped countries play a prestigious role in the health care team of the hospital.

During the last few years, laboratory examination became an important part of diagnosis and integral units of hospitals. Aseptic surgry, X-ray examination, MRI and microscopic techniques have made hospital safe. Anesthesia and psychotherapeutics became specialized and professional. Hospital became organisation for diagnosis and treatment for rich and poor patients. Hospitals were modernized by philanthropic learning of society and the welfare programmes of the government. At present hospitals cover the therapeutic and preventive aspects for health care considering need of community. The primary emphasis is placed on the care of bed ptients. Hospitals also care the potentially sick persons in their normal living situation. They have been assuming more and more responsibilty for programmes of preventive medicine. They serve as a medium for improvement of the public health.

Present status

The Hospital provides special facilities and trained personnel to facilitate the work of the physician in his primary position for taking care of the patient. The physician is the focal point about all activities of the hospital revolves. In the delivery of medical services to the patients, the medical specialists, nurses, pharmacists, dieticians, etc became a most important factor. The hospital facilities are advanced continuously according to changes and advances in medical science. A modern hospital lowers the incidence of disease through early detection and treatment. Medical science is advanced by forming links between the general public and policy makers. Bigger hospital co-operate to smaller hospitals. There is coordination between specialized hospitals and general hospitals. Private hospitals co-operate with public hospitals. The whole system is integrated for the welfare of general persons. Doctors and nurses are trained in colleges attached to hospitals. Apollo hospitals with over 8000 beds in more than 41 hospitals, a string of nursing and hospital management colleges and dual lifelines of pharmacies and diagnostic clinics providing a safety net across Asia. At Apollo hospitals, there are exceptional good clinical success rates and superior technology with comfort.

A teaching hospital is one which is used extensively for the clinical instruction of medical students. A minor teaching hospital is used only for a limited amount of student instruction, such as occasional demonstration or clinics.

Traditionally, teaching hospitals are places where the new medical graduates seek postgraduate training. They undergo one year of hospital training as an intern. They spend two or more additional years in a hospital as a resident in some specialty, such as internal medicine, surgery, pediatrics or radiology. On the other hand, some community hospitals maintain intern and residency programmes.

Most of the young fresh physician preferred to work in teaching hospital because they assure them for the contemporary educational opportunities coupled with broad experiences in the clinical case of patients, teaching and research.

Air ambulance concept: Airlifting patients or doctors in emergency cases – is a concept fast catching up in the sophisticated Hospital in the country. Kokilaben Dhirubhai Ambani hospital, in Mumbai, is the latest to have this facility. The hospital, scheduled to be commissioned by early 2007, is planning to introduce the service in collaboration with a leading aviation company. The multi-specialty hospital will have a helipad on its terrace to ferry patients in the case of emergency.

Escort Hospitals in New Delhi recently renovated its facility with a helipad on its rooftop and became the first hospital in the country to offer this service to its high-profile patients. It now plans to tie up with Deccan Aviation, a subsidiary of low-cost carrier Air Deccan, to fly air ambulance as an integral part of the package of services which patients can avail of.

Manipal hospital in Bangalore, too, is readying to launch this service in association with an airline company. In Mumbai, a couple of other hospitals, including the proposed multi-specialty hospitals of the Apollo group, are planning helipads at their complexes.

Industry also recognizes the importance of teaching hospital by virtue of the special coverage it receives from the company's medical service representatives as well as its desire to financially support both educational and research programmes.

Classification of Hospitals

There are different ways to classify hospitals. A single hospital may fall into more than one class. Broadly, the hospitals are classified on the basis of clinical, non clinical and medicinal hospital, and on the basis of size and cost.

1. Clinical Hospitals

This type of classification is depndent on the basis of diagnosis and treatment. It is further subdivided on the basis of speiality and length of stay.

(i) **Medicine :** Medicine for general communicable diseases and specialized medicines for psychiatric (nervous) disorders, tuberculosis, leprosy, asthma, cancer, etc.

(ii) **Surgery :** Surgery is performed for the orthopedic, gynecologic (for female) and otolarygologic patients.

(iii) **Maternilty :** This type of hospital deals with the delivery cases.

(iv) **Paediatric :** Hospitals treating the diseases of children.

On the basis of length of stay, a hospital may provide short term stay (less than 30 days), long term stay (more than 30 days in case of chronic diseases) and custodial stay (for psychiatric and mentally retarded patients).

2. Non-clinical Hospitals

This type of classification is dependent on the ownership of hospitals which may be of two types.

(i) **Public ownership :** Public hspitals my be governed by the :

(a) **Central Government :** Like railway hospital, defence hospitals, All India Institute of Medical Sciences, New Delhi, P.G. Institute of Medical Sciences at Pondicherry, Lucknow and Chandigarh.

(b) **State Government :** Like civil hospital at district headquaters, Sasson hospital in Pune and J.J hospital in Mumbai.

(c) **Local Self government :** These hospitals are run by municipalities or corporatios like NDMC hospital in Delhi;

Kasturba hospital run by MCD in Delhi; BMC Hospital and Bhagwati Hospital in Mumbai.

(ii) **Pivate ownership :** They are run by the following types of organizations :

(a) **Trusts :** The board of trustees manage the affairs e.g. Bombay hospital (Mumbai), Jaslok hospital (Mumbai).

(b) **Religious bodies :** Christian Medical College Hospital (Vellore & Ludihiana), Ram Krishna Mission Hospital (Calcutta).

(c) **Limited companies :** They are governed by public limited companies, where the public subscribes to the shares e.g. Medinova centres (Baroda), Apollo Hospital Ltd. (Chennai and Delhi), Escorts Heart Research Institute and Hospital (Delhi), Modi Hospital (Delhi).

3. Medicinal based hospitals

These hospitals are :

(i) **Allopathic Hospitals** e.g. Ram Manohar Lohia Hospital, New Delhi.

(ii) **Ayurvedic Hospitals** in Jammu and Trivendrum, e.g., Amba Ayurveda Hospital, Kottayam in Kerala.

(iii) **Homeopathic Hospitals :** Nehru Homeopathic Hospital (Delhi).

(iv) **Unani Hospital** e.g. Hamdard Dawakhana (Delhi), Unani Dawakha (Aligarh).

(v) **Naturalpathy (Yoga) Hospitals** e.g. hospitals running at Lucknow (UP), Pune, Kerala, and Karnataka.

4. Size base Hospitals

Hospitals can be classified on the basis of size :

(a) **Large hospitals** (beds 1000 and more) e.g. J.J. Group of Hospitals in Mumbai have an intake of 1400 beds; K.E.M. Mumbai has 1600 beds. Other large hospitals are AIIMS (Delhi), Safdarjung Hospital (Delhi), G.T.B Hospital (Delhi).

(b) **Medium hospital** (beds between 500-1000 beds) e.g. Bombay Hospital, Jaslok Hospital.

(c) **Small hospital** (beds between 100-500) e.g. Beach Candy Hospital (Delhi), Jaipur Golden Hospital (Delhi), Majeedia Hospital (Delhi).

(d) **Very small hospital**-(beds less than 100).

5. Cost based Hospitals

(a) **Elite hospitals :** Jaslok and Hinduja are run for the privilage. They are a symbol of high tech medical development. The rooms rates vay between Rs. 1500-3000 per day. The deluxe rooms are equppied with refrigerator, TV, and telephone. Excepting the medical care, they are like five star hotels. They are therefore, often called five star hospitals. But even these elite institutions reserve a particular percentage of their capacity for the poorer sections and subsidise a particular percentage of their accommodation. Jaslok Hospital, Batra Hospital, Jaipur Golden Hospital, etc has reserved have reserved a particular percentage to the poor patients. Apollo Hospital, Escort Hospital, Batra Hospital are also high cost hospitals.

(b) **Budget hospitals :** These are meant for moderate budget and low budget users, e.g. Civil Hospital, Corporation Hospitals.

(c) **Private Hospitals/Nursing Homes :** These medical centres are operated generally in all the metropolitan cities and towns in India by either a single or group of private practitioners or husband-wife team. They are proprietary or partnership concern, general nursing homes, with facilities for general surgery. Some nursing homes are specialised for cardiac, paediatric or opthalmological. The treatment cost of nursing homes are generally very high and sometime irrational. Therefore, there is a demand to regulate the private nursing homes by suitable enactment.

(d) **Teaching Hospitals :** Hospitals can be teaching or research centres to which a medical college is attached. They can be integrated hospitals where many medical and surgical departments are integrated or alternaive systems of medicine are integrated. The All India Institute of Medical Science, New Delhi; GTB hospital, Delhi, PGI, Chandigarh; J.N. College, Aligarh, etc. are teaching hospitals.

There are in-plant hospitals run as a part of of bussiness organization for the health care of its employee and immediate community surrounding it. There is no system of accreditation for hospitals here in India as it prevails in other advanced countries. The time has come how to take steps for rating of hospitals on the criteria of service quality, service availability, patient satisfaction and perceived image.

2

Chapter

Hospital Organisation

The infrastructure of hospital organization is identical to that of an industrial plant; only the difference is of nomenclature of position. For example, the Director or Administrator of a hospital may be the General Manager of an industry. Less administrative position are needed in a smaller hospital. Private hospitals are organized by a corporation or board of trustees. Government hospitals usually managed by a board of trustees but no corporate body.

Basic Concept of Hospital Organization

The successful hospital is based upon good community oriented planning, good design and construction and good administration. A progressive hospital will build its services on certain knowledge of the community it is to serve. Organisation is a process of achieving the objectives by grouping people in order to get the work done. The ultimate aim of the hospital is to provide optimum health care. Its organization is based upon the following principles :

1. **Team co-ordination :** An individual supervices a professional team of medical/paramedical staff. The services are integrated and coordinated.
2. **Division of services :** An observer looks after the working system. Activities analysis is an important decision to shape the organisation. Hospital undertakes a number of activities– diagnostic, treatment or therapy, rehabilitation, education and prevention. These activities are further sub-classified. Groups and sub-groups are formed to carry out these activities. The whole

work load is divided into manageable units of health services. Each unit contributes to the total spectrum of health services.

3. **Homogenous approach :** A hospital caters to both ambulatory and bed patients (out-patients and in-patients). The organisation should form a homogenous approach with common or integrated services.
4. **Evaluation of services :** Services provided by the hospital should be rated in terms of quality and adequacy for meeting the patient's and community requirements.
5. **Administrative responsibility :** The relations amongst the various people and tasks in a hospital must be carefully maintained. Responsibility should be assigned appropriately. Once responsibility is assigned, accountability should be reported to the superior for its performance. This is necessary to ensure a high quality of patient care.
6. **Budget preparation and financing :** Large hospitals treat almost 15 lacs patient per year and perform 18 thousand major surgeries and 33 thousand minor surgeries. Their yearly budget is about Rs. 30-35 crores. Many hospitals have their own finance. The hospitals should, therefore, design an effective organization and techniques to optimise their resources. There should be budgeting and a planned programme for capital financing.
7. **Talent search :** A hospital should be staffed by competent medical experts and non-medical staff. The organisation should formulate a programme to attract good physicians and surgical specialists as well as to attach the patients.
8. **Governing body :** Each hospital has the top management to decide its course of action, and policy guidelines and to exercise overall supervision and control. It is the legal and moral responsibility for the conduct of hospital as an institution. It is accountable to the patient staff community and the sponsoring organisation.

Organisational Pattern of a Typical Hospital

A hospital is maintained for the purpose of health care of the patients. The functional department of clinical services is the most important division of a hospital which needs supportive services like pharmacy and nursing, and administrative support of office. Appropriate pharmacy, nursing and administrative units are commonly found in all hospitals. The hospitals needs maintenance and safety. It should have sound house-keeping and maintenance heads.

The top-management of hospital is responsible for its overall policies and control. It is constituted by the governing board and the administrator. The administrator is the Chief Executive or Director of the hospital. The heads of individual services are responsible to the administrator.

A hospital administrative organisation has the following administrative pattern :

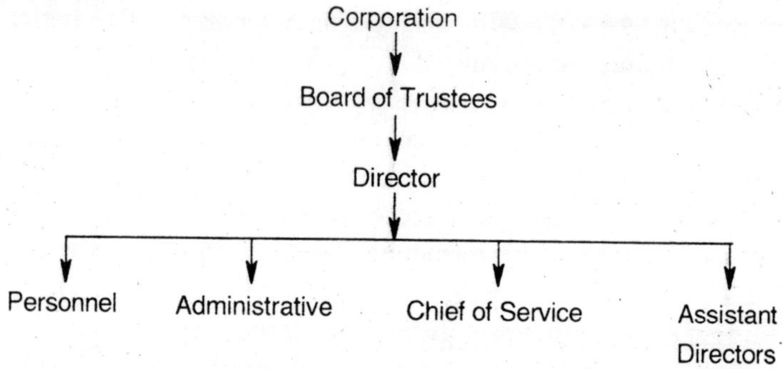

The duties of Assistant Directors are sub-divided as follows :

(a) **Assistant Director Professional Services :** He control the ambulatory service, administration, dialysis of kidney transplant unit, dietary service, employee health clinic, house staff, medical records, physiotherapy, social service, respiratory therapy.

(b) **Assistant Director Special Services :** He control the blood bank, data processing, communications, pharmacy, laboratory control, laboratory clinical research, radiology, radiotherapy, pathology, safety engineering, system engineering.

(c) **Associate Director Nursing :** He/She is responsible for nursing service, ambulatory, speciality units, operating room, pavilions, staff education, unit management, school of nursing.

(d) **Associate Director Finance :** He is responsible for accounting, credit collections, admitting, grants and contracts, treasurer's office, purchasing and stores, insurances, audit.

(e) **Assistant Director of Development :** He is responsible for chaplaincy service, public relations, volunteers, secretary of the corporation.

(f) **Assistant Director of Plant Service :** He is responsible for engineering, house keeping, linen laundry, escort and messenger, security, parking, transport.

(g) **Assistant Director Community Medical Service :** He is responsible for home care programme, nursing home liasion, model cities, emergency ward.

Hospital organisation typically consists of following divisions.

1. Management or Governing Body

Each hospital has an organized governing body. The legal status of a hospital is maintained by a society, a trust or a company; named as board of trustees, board of governors, borad of directors or commissioners, etc.

(a) Objectives of the Governing Body

1. The governing body is responsible for the functioning of a hospital providing high quality patient care.
2. It is also responsible for moderanisation of available facilities to improve the quality of health care.
3. The interpretation of standard, should be simplified and clarified to remove all possible ambiguities and confusions.

(b) Composition of Governing Body

A corporation consists of a large number of people from widely scattered areas. A representative group, from within the corporation membership, is elected to a board of trustees. This group is also known as the board of governors, board of managers or board of directors.

Generally, the above board includes a representation from the community served by the hospital and its members are selected for their ability to contribute to its effective management.

It is required by state laws that the governing body adopts by-laws identifying the purposes of the hospital and the means of fulfilling them. Included in the by-laws are the following :

(i) definition of the powers and duties of the governing body officers, committees and chief executive office.

(ii) qualifications for governing body members.

(iii) method of selection of membership.

(iv) committees – kinds, appointment and membership tenure.

The by-laws also describe the authority delegated to the Chief Executive Officer (Director or Administrator) and to the medical staff, such a delegation of authority does not preclude the governing body from exercising the control and authority required to meet its responsibility for the conduct of the hospital. The governing body always has the right to rescind or cancel any such delegation.

As part of the organizational process, the governing body elects its officers and appoints a wide variety of committees necessary for the discharge of their duties. These may include an Executive Committee, Building Committee, Investment Finance Committee and a Joint Confusions Committee.

(c) Duties of Governing Body

1. There shall be full disclosure of hospital ownership and control.
2. The governing body shall adopt by-laws in accordance with legal requirements and its responsibility to the community.
3. The governing body shall provide a procedure for the selection of its officers, adopt a schedule of meetings, and define attendance requirements and the method of documenting governing body proceedings.
4. Governing body members shall be selected, unless otherwise provided by law, in accordance with the hospital's by-laws and, if applicable, articles of incorporation or charter.
5. The governing body shall provide mechanisms for fulfilling the functions necessary to the discharge of its responsibilities.
6. The governing body shall require that the medical staff establish mechanisms designed to assure the achievement and maintenance of high standards of medical practice and patient care.
7. The governing body shall provide for institutional planning to meet the health needs of the community.
8. The governing body shall appoint a chief executive officer whose qualifications, responsibilities, authority, and accountability shall be defined in writing.
9. The medical staff by-laws, rules and regulations shall be subject to governing body approval. This approval shall not be unreasonably withheld.
10. The governing body shall hold the medical staff responsible for making recommendations concerning initial medical staff appointments, reappointments, termination of appointments, the delineation of clinical privileges, and the curtailment of clinical privileges.

(d) Sub Committees

The governing body will also constitute various committees for proper functioning which may be ad-hoc or standing committees.

(i) *Executive Committee* : It takes decisions to form adhoc committees and task committees. It acts autocratically in emergencies. It reviews specific and board reports before final ratification by the full board. It also reviews other committee reports.

(ii) *Joint Conference Committee* : It is a combination of the representatives of Board and the clinical services, with the administrator acting as its secretary. It is liaison committee.

(iii) *Professional Committee* : It is responsible to the executive committee. It is made up of selected Board members who study and make recommendations on all dimensions of clinical services. They work closely with the medical staff and administration. Their aim is to be upgrade the quality of health care.

(iv) *Finance Committee* : It reviews the budget planning, financial statements and related problems.

(v) *Other Committee* : Some temporary and some permanent. They are formed depending upon the need and situation. These include buildings, public relations (PR) and others.

The administrator usually serves as an ex-office member of all committees of the Board and should attend all the meetings.

2. Administration

The active management of hospital includes the board of trustees who select the administrator and his associate staff, assistant supervisors and department heads.

The hospital administrator must know and understand his community, its people, their historical traditions, the value structure that is at work, the resources available, and the weakness to be reckoned with any course of action. Armed with this knowledge and understanding, he must educate the employees for the enterprise, its goals, its problems, its needs, and its opportunities for contribution to the community.

Responsibilities of an Administrator : The modern hospital administrator should be a specialist in administration, an educator, a community adviser and an organiser. Reporting to the governing body, he has responsibility for the operation of the entire institution, assuring the medical and scientific staffs, the trustees and the patients of the highest possible standards of both service and economy. The future of the institution depends, in significant measure, on the vision of the hospital administrator.

The main function of the administrator is to enforce trustee policy in the daily management routine. In addition, he is required to take all reasonable steps to assure that the hospital complies with applicable laws and regulations; establish an organisational structure to carry out the programmes of the hospital and to meet the needs of the patients; to implement the governing body policy on the financial management of the hospital; and to develop and implement a comprehensive management reporting system throughout the hospital.

The administrator is a link between the Board and the clinical services and between the Board and all other employees. The administrator's job is onerous and requires delegation of matching authority to carry out his heavy responsibilities. The administrator attends the meetings of the governing body. He frames the overall administrative policies. He is privileged to attend the meetings of medical staff. The administrator is empowered to modify the internal organisation of the hospital in response to current operating conditions. He is incharge of the admission and discharge of all patients. He does not interfere in the clinical activities of the hospital, but brings the lapses in conforming to overall policy of the hospital to the notice of chief of staff. The administrator is a link between the Board and the employees. The administrator ensures the compliance of legal formalities. He oversees the training of interns, student nurses, volunteers and auxiliary workers. He ensures smooth running of the outpatient department.

These days training programmes are available at several institutes in hospital administration. There are full-fledged post-graduate management courses in the discipline. Mostly persons with basic degree in science or medicine or pharmacy, followed by course in hospital administration are preferred these days for the job of administrator. To be successful he must not have only administrative ability, but an appreciation of clinical environment in which he has to practice, and an overall compassionate attitude.

The administrator has to provide facilities, equipment and assistance so that the patient is restored to health completely.

The administrator exercises his personnel management powers of staffing and directing in constitution with the department heads. He is responsible to provide the employees a conductive work environment.

The administrator prepares a budget for approval by the Governing Board.

The administrator is responsible to coordinate with other institutions, and enriches his own institution by borrowing ideas from others and organises his own staff to develop relations with other institutions.

3. Medical Staff

A medical staff is responsible for the quality of all medical care provided to patients and for the ethical conduct and professional practices.

Generally, medical staff membership is limited to individuals who are fully licensed to practice medicine or dentistry. As a body, this group usually organises itself to provide for the election or appointment of officers and committees whose function is to create and maintain an optimal level of professional performance.

The framework of the medical staff will vary from hospital to hospital due to varying size and activities of the hospital and the staff. However, the staff may be divided into the following categories: active medical staff; associate medical staff; courtesy medical staff; consulting medical staff and honorary medical staff.

The active medical staff is responsible for the delivery of the preponderance of medical service within the hospital and is most involved in the organisational and administrative duties pertaining to the medical staff.

The associate medical staff consists of individuals who are being considered for advancement to the active medical staff. These practitioners are appointed and assigned to the various services in the same manner as are members of the active medical staff.

The courtesy medical staff consists of practitioners who are eligible for staff membership, who are given privileges to admit an occasional patient to the hospital. Courtesy staff members may neither vote nor hold office in the medical staff organisation.

The consulting medical staff consists of medical practitioners of recognised professional ability who are not members of the preceding categories of staff membership.

The honorary medical staff consists of former staff members, retired or emeritus, and of other practitioners whom the medical staff chooses to honour.

4. Clinical Divisions

The degree of departmentalisation of the clinical divisions depends upon the degree of specialisation of the medical staff. In small communities, there are two major departments in a hospital – medicine and surgery. Supportive services such as radiology and pathology are also offered but are generally limited in their capability to provide service. In those areas where there are two or more small hospitals, it is common to have a single department of pathology or radiology servicing both institutions. However, in the large metropolitan areas the hospital staff is highly specialised and, therefore, there are greater subdivisions within a particular department.

Generally, the department of medicine includes the following subdivisions :

Internal medicine
Cardiology
Infectious diseases
Dermatology
Endocrinology
Geriatrics
Immunology
Allergy
Gastroenterology
Nephrology
Neurology
Psychiatry
Pulmonary Diseases
Rheumatology
Pediatrics

The department of energy is generally divided into the following sub-divisions :

General surgery
Orthopedic surgery
Neurologic and Gynecology
Ophthalmology
Dental and Oral surgery
Otolaryngology
Plastic Surgery
Thoracic Surgery
Urology

In addition there may be a division of general practice as well as a division of physical medicine and rehabilitation within the hospital.

Clinical Services

No hospital successful without its medical staff. They make the success of the hospital. High clinical standards are the goal of any hospital.

The medical staff of a hospital is an organised body of physicians and dentists. The medical staff of a hospital is an organised body of physicians and dentists. The medical staff has a three-fold responsibility: (1) to the patient, (2) to the hospital, and (3) to the medical staff's by laws. The positions are filled by appointment by the governing body or by election amongst themselves. There is a formal relationship between the medical staff and the administrator, and preferably it occurs at the level of executive committee. One physician is designated as chief of staff by the governing body. The appointment is tenured for a year or for more than one year. His clinical acumen is remarkable and coupled with administrative ability. He works closely with the administrator and other departmental heads. The administrator has full control over purely administrative matters but the chief of staff has full control over clinical matters. There are many overlapping areas, in which they have to show a mutual understanding. The chief of staff is responsible for the smooth functioning of the clinical services, and supervises the clinical work done. He may be given a deputy, called assistant, chief of staff.

Department Heads

In a large hospital, there are departments of pharmacy, nursing, central supply, office administration, maintenance and several clinical specia-lities. Competent chiefs or heads of each of these departments are designated, in consultation with the medical staff. Mostly, large hospital prefers salaried full-time professional departmental heads or chiefs. His functions are as follows :

1. He is responsible for the overall running of the department and the quality of service rendered.
2. He is a member of the executive committee and a member of committees in his department.
3. He is responsible for submission departmental progress report to the medical staff, administrator and the board.
4. He is responsible for educational programmes in his department.
5. If he heads a medical department, he is responsible for the professional care of the patients also.
6. He recommends the qualifications of other staff members of his department.

The major departments in a hospital are as follows :

General medical department : It is basic to any clinical activity and departmented according to specialities – general diagnosis, therapy, general, medical and nursing care, paediatrics, psychiatry, neurology, cardiology, dermatology, pathology, laboratory, mental hygiene, physical medicine, urology, communicable diseases, therapy and complications of surgery, obstetrics, gynaecology, ENT conditions and orthopaedics. Allergy, gland, respiratory, gastrointestinal, gerinatrics, chronic diseases and clinical research are also parts of general medical services.

Paediatrics, physical medicine, rehabilative services and medical social services are important areas of patient care these days.

Surgical department : Most of the patients admitted to the hospital for major or minor operation. Functions of the surgical department are the same as for other clinical services – prevention, diagnosis, therapy, restoration, research and education. Larger hospitals use full-time salaried chiefs of clinical departments. Professionally trained and experienced surgeons are given full surgical privileges, and those who get sufficient experience under them might be given limited surgical privileges. Qualified physicians serve as first assistants during surgery, while nurses and aides serve as second and third assistants. The operating room nursing supervisor directs the nursing staff and is responsible to the director of nursing services functionally and to chief of the surgical staff administratively. In most of the hospitals, there are the departments of anaesthesiologist. The overall responsibility is, however, of the Chief of surgery and the Chief of maternity services. The recovery after surgery is an area that is receiving attention. The physical facilities for operating room requires careful planning and equipping. Till recently, the central services department is the focal point for processing, sterilizing and dispensing practically all operational equipment and supplies. The central department also acts as the central distribution centre for the pharmacy and hospital store room. It had close interface with the surgical services. However, these days the pharmacy services have emerged as a separate department, and supplies such vitally essential commodities as large volume intravenous fluids.

Maternity department : Hospital deliveries have been accepted now all over. There should be good planning for the number of maturity beds. Maternity care includes considerations of staffing including nursing staffing, maternity unit procedures, delivery unit procedures, hospital records, new-born infant care, identification of infants, premature infant services, infant feeding, infant records, etc.

Pathology and Clinical Laboratory Department : The practice of medicine in these days is dependent upon more and more laboratory examinations to facilitate correct diagnosis, treatment and prevention of diseases. Some diseases are diagnosed on the basis of laboratory reports, e.g. diabetes, syphilis, blood diseases, etc. Some diseases can be diagnosed earlier due to laboratory facilities, e.g. tuberculosis, cancer. The control and treatment of some diseases are added by the laboratory, e.g. anaemia and infectious diseases. The laboratory reports help surgical practice, e.g. urine analysis, Rh-typing, blood typing, post-operative tests, etc.

Necropsies are an important part of medical education. The laboratory works under a qualified pathologist who is assisted by a number of medical technicians. They have to keep in mind the workload, staffing, and routine tests while organising this department. Blood bank is managed by a hospital committee of which pathologist is a member who looks after the proper use of blood and its derivatives in the hospital. A proper procedure is laid down for requesting laboratory examination. The design of laboratory forms and records demand keen attention. The laboratory examinations are charged for each test or at a flat rate, or at a graded flat rate or by a point system with a sliding schedule of unit charges. Physical facilities of a laboratory require careful planning. There is generally a modular arrangement. The typical installation includes :

1. Haemotology/blood bank unit
2. Urine analysis unit
3. Biochemistry unit
4. Histology unit
5. Serology-Bacteriology unit

The administrative area provides space for waiting room, vein puncture cubicle for drawing blood specimens, specimen toilt, basal-metabolism/ECG room and pathologist's office. The auxiliary service area provides for glass washing and sterilizing units. The laboratory should be well-equipped with modern equipments. This department also administers the morgue, if the hospital has more than 50 beds. It should have enough mortuary refrigeration capacity. Exhaust ventilation is necessary in morgue area. In better hospitals, there are separate facilities for morgue and necropsy.

Radiological department : Radiology is the diagnostic and therapeutic arm of the hospital. This service is placed under the direction of a competent radiologist. This department uses radiography and fluoroscopy. The radiologist is responsible to the Chief of Staff for clinical policies and activities and to the administrator for administrative aspects. He is assisted by technologists. Physical facilities of radiology department should be properly planned.

Dental Department : Every hospital should offer at least the minimum in dental services, especially to care for emergencies. The dental services are organised into sections to conform to the areas of recognised dental specialities. The department is placed under chief of dental services. Generally, the dental services include : (a) dentistry for children, (b) dental X-rays, (c) oral hygiene, (d) oral pathology, (e) oral surgery, (f) periodontics, (g) restorative dentistry and (h) cosmetic dentistry.

Intensive Care Unit : The Intensive Care Unit (ICU) or special care unit is a special facility set up by most hospitals in order to care for the critically ill or injured. It has equipment to treat any possible emergency and is staffed by specially trained nurses and doctors. Some hospitals have special ICU's devoted to the care of parties who have suffered from a heart attack or a serious burn. These are known as coronary care units or burn units.

Due to its unique nature, daily charges for confinement in an ICU unit are usually significantly higher than the charges for a semi-private room where most patients stay. In view of the extra expense and necessity involved with this type of care, medical plans often provide higher benefits for ICU's than that allowed for the semiprivate room.

5. Supporting Divisions

To those unfamiliar with the hospital environment, it would appear that the hospital consists of the clinical departments only. Actually, the clinical departments would not be able to function without the supporting services. Amongst the supporting services are the nursing department, the dietary service, laboratory services, the medical records department, the blood bank, the central sterile supply and the soial service department.

6. Nursing Division

Nursing has not only impact on mechanical practice but also on other divisions in hospital. The nursing team, made up of workers with varying degrees of nursing skill and directed by a professional nurse, now replaces the single nurse who once did everything for the patient. Today's nursing practitioner recognises social, psychological or religious problems with the patient that might influence his physical well being and refer those that lie outside the province of nursing to the person, most competent to deal with them. Helping the patients to themselves is another new element of nursing practice, because of increased emphasis on self care by the patient is an aid to early recovery. The new patterns of nursing service thus brought about are often misunderstood by the public when the changes are the reasons behind them are not explained. Thus in 1964, the National League for Nursing directed a statement concerning the basic assumptions which one could made about nursing care in various aspects of nursing service as a means of improving service wherever it is given. The following are the basic assumptions of nursing care :

(a) Nursing care encompasses health promotion, the care and prevention of disease or disability, rehabilitation, teaching, counselling and emotional support as well as the care of illness.

(b) Nursing care is an integral part of total health care and is planned and administered in combination with related medical, educational and welfare services.

(c) Nursing personnels respect individuality, dignity and rights of every person, regardless of race, colour, creed, national origin, social or economic status.

The nursing service is organised similarly to any other large service in the hospital. There is at least a Head of Director of Nursing who is generally an experienced nurse with administrative talent. The administrative nursing services carries ultimate administrative authority and responsibility in one or more health facilities for the nursing services provided individuals and families.

7. Dietectic Division

An essential service of each institution is that of the dietary department. The dietetic service should be organised in such a manner that it shall effectively apply the principles of the science of nutrition to the preparation of palatable and appropriate food. The services are generally directed by a qualified person and staffed by adequate numbers of dietitians and technical and clerical personnel. Qualified personnel in the dietary and division are generally considered to be individuals who are registered or have met that Association's standards for qualification.

In addition to the purchasing, planning and preparation of menus, both for patients and employees, the dietitian is generally responsible for recording dietary histories of patients such as those with food allergies and those unable to accept a limited diet regimen, interviewing patients regarding their food habits, counselling patients and their families concerning normal or modified regimens, and encouraging patients to participate in planning their own normal or modified regimens, and participating in appropriate ward rounds and conferences.

8. Medical Records Division

Every hospital is required by law to maintain adequate medical records of their patients. These must be accurately documented, readily accessible and can be easily used for retrieving and compiling information.

The purposes of the medical record are :

(a) to serve as a basis for planning and for continuity of patient care.

(b) to provide a means of communication among the physician and any professionals contributing to the patient's care.

(c) To furnish documentary evidence for the course of the patient's illness and treatment during each hospital stay.

(d) To serve as a basis for review, study and evaluation of the care rendered to the patient.

(e) To assist in protecting the legal interest of the patient, hospital and responsible practitioner.

(f) To provide data for use in research and education.

The medical record must contain all significant informations and should be sufficiently detailed to enable another practitioner to assume the care of the patient at any time, a consultant to give an opinion after his examination of the patient and the practitioner to give effective continuing care to the patient.

9. Medical Social Service Division

The Medical Social Service Department is an important liaison between the hospital and the patient and his community. The qualified social worker represents a discipline whose main professional focus is on the social aspects of the patient and his family. Social service personnel generally provide information relating to medical social study of appropriate patients, social therapy and rehabilitation of patients, home environmental investigations for attending physician, cooperative activities with community agencies, social service summaries, and follow-up reports of discharged patients, confirming disposition, when obtained.

10. Anaesthesia Division

The Anaesthesia Service of a hospital is generally directed by a physician member of the medical staff who has had special training and is responsible for the following: quality of anaesthesia care rendered by anaesthetist in the surgical and obstetrical areas, availability of equipment necessary for administering anaesthesia and for related resuscitative effect, development of regulations concerning anaesthetic safety and retrospective evaluation of all anaesthesia care.

Anaesthesia care is usually provided by anaesthesiologists, other qualified physician anaesthetist, qualified nurse anaesthetist, or appropriately supervised trainees in an approved education programme. Whenever nurse anaesthetists are employed, they generally provide general anaesthesia under the overall direction of the departmental director.

11. Pharmacy Division

Althouth the pharmacy department is only one of the many divisions of a hospital, it exerts a great deal of influence on the professional stature of the hospital as well as upon the economics of the total operational costs of the institution because of its inter-relation with and the inter-dependency of other services upon it.

In the community practice of pharmacy, the pharmacist is keenly aware of the doctor-patient-pharmacist relationship. In this setting, the doctor diagnoses and prescribes, the pharmacist dispenses the medication and the patient administers the prescribed drug to himself or at most it is administered to him, under ordinary circumstances, by a member of his family.

This is not true in the hospital or in an extended care facility. In this setting we find coordination among the doctor-pharmacist-patient and the professional nurse who assumes the major responsibility of administering all medications to the patient (unless the patient is on a self-medication regimen).

Clearly then, the pharmacist who practices his profession in an institutional environment must be aware of the forces operating around him, and he must learn not only to understand them, but to assist in marshalling them towards the ultimate goal of better patient care.

The function of hospital pharmacy begins with the procurement of drugs and end with their distribution in patients. It continues to play a role even after administration of by instituting a prepare drug delivery information system.

Hospital pharmacy generally has a manufacturing extension and a medical stores. There are sub-functions of sterilisation and quality control.

Hospital pharmacy head is on an equal footing with other departmental heads, and is responsible to the administrator. He renders a professional service to the medical and the nursing staffs. He is responsible for purchase and supplies of drugs. He is a member of therapeutics committee which adopts a suitable hospital formulary.

Hospital pharmacy brings about a redefinition of the usual roles played by the physicians outside the hospital setting. Here, inside a hospital as a part of the triad of the physician-nurse-pharmacist, the physician restricts himself to diagnosis and prescription. The nurse takes over from here, and administers the drugs which she receives from the pharmacist who either makes and dispense the drugs.

12. House-Keeping

Good house-keeping in an invaluable part of any hospital. The task of house-keeping facilities is carried out by the other departments. Generally, it is carried out by the house-keeper, who heads his department. House-keeper is well versed in home economics and principles of physican sciences. He/She is aware of the characteristics and qualities of soaps, detergents, cleaning agents, their selection and use. He/she handles many unskilled workers who are continuously trained. Some of the important aspects of house keeping are cleaning, dusting, waxing, moping, washing of walls, bed making, general sanitation and linen services etc.

13. Financial Resources of Hospital

The financial resources of a hospital play a significant role and exercise influence on every patient, employees, trustees and the people who avail of services offered by the hospital. A pharmacist must have a clear idea about the ways and means for managing the available hospital finance. The following are some important financial resources on a hospital.

1. The charges received frcm the patients against the hospital bills, which included registration charges, tests room doctor's fee and medicines, etc.
2. The bills or charges received by the patients are either fully paid by himself or full or a part of payment is made by a third party such as government hospitals, central governments health schemes or employees health insurance scheme, etc.
3. Income received from invested funds.
4. Income which is derived from overhead charges or research projects carried out in hospitals, etc.
5. Donations received from individual or various organisations.

HEALTH DELIVERY SYSTEM IN INDIA

After independence, India has made considerable progress in economic and social development. India has invested huge sums of money in development of extensive health delivery system which caters to a population of 1000 million resising in 6,00,000 villages.

India compared to other developing nations spends slightly higher amount in the health system. It spends 6% of GDP or $13 per capita in the health sector. However, many of the key health indicators are very low, communicable diseases continue to be major problem, material mortality is high and morbidity especially among the poor enacts a high toll.

At the Central Government level, there is the Union Ministry of Health and the Family Welfare which is a apex organisation. The Central Ministry formulates the overall health policy and plans the new health schemes. It gives total support for national programs and runs Central Government Health Services (CGHS) for Central Government employees. It also offers financial assistance to the State Governments. The organisation of health at the Central Government level is illustrated diagramatically here.

Organisation of Health Delivery System at the Centre Level

Union Health Minister
Union Ministry of Health and Family Welfare

Minister of State for Health
↓
Secretary staff

Ministry of Health and Family Welfare
↓
Secretarial staff (Secretory, Additional Secretory. Joint Secretory, drawn from Indiian Civil Services)
↓
Commissioner
↓
Dy. Commissioners
↓
Secretaries
↓
Regional Directors
↓
Director General of Health Services (DGHS)
↓
Additional DGHS

↓

Dy. Director of Health Services for Medical care and Hospitals
↓
1. Health Admn. for :
   (a) International health
   (b) Medical care in hospitals
2. Medical and Professional Education
3. Fellowships

Dy. Director for Health Services : Public Health
↓
1. Public Health
2. Health Education
3. National Malaria Eradication Programme
4. Communicable diseases

Dy. Director for Health Services Gen. Admn.
↓
1. Central Admn. Civil Service
2. Supplies
3. Transport
4. Workshops etc.

Organisation of Health and Delivery System at State Government Level

The administrative units take care for health administration in rural and urban areas. The director of health is the single administrative officer, who is assisted by several assistants/deputies in various programmes.

The following chart illustrates this :

State Health Minister Ministry of Health
↓
Deputy Minister
↓
Health Secretariat
↓
Director of Health Services
↓
Dy. Director of Health Services
↓

ADHS (Medical Education)	ADHS (Nursing)	ADHS (MCH)	ADHS (Family Welfare)	ADHS (Nutrition)	ADHS (School Health) Centres)	ADHS (Primary Health	ADHS (Health Education)

A Chief Medical Officer (CMO) is responsible for hospital administration and for community health work. Chief Medical Officer is responsible for all government hospitals, taluka hospitals and jail hospitals in the district. In many states, there is a separate officer, called District Health Officer (DHO), responsible for supervisions of health services in municipal areas and blòck areas including primary health centres.

Primary Health Centres (PHC)

These cater to the health care of the rural areas. They are not self-sufficient. They depend upon the facilities provided by civil hospital (District HQ Hospital) or Taluka Hospital. Family welfare activities are now assigned to family welfare centre, attached to PHC. The staffing pattern of a PHC is as :

Medical Officer (1), Block Extension Educator (1), Pharmacist (1), Family Welfare field workers (3), Accountant-cum-clerk (1), Auxillary Nurse, Midwife (4), Health Visitor (1) and Female Assistant (7).

3
Chapter

Hospital Pharmacy

The Hospital Pharmacy is a department in which the drugs are procured/manufactured, stored, compounded, check for quality, dispensed, packed and distributed to in-patients and out-patients by competent and legally qualified pharmacists. It is an important department which caters the need of physicians, nurses, technician and other staff members of Hospital. Modern system of Hospital Pharmacy also provides drug information and drug monitoring services. Today, the practice of Hospital Pharmacy encompasses a wide array of roles and responsibilities, including the very important task of increasing accessibility to accurate and ethical information on medicines use and pharmacotherapy in and outside the hospital setting, including epidemics and emergency situations.

Functions of Hospital Pharmacy

Hospital Pharmacy Services offers expertise in both clinical service and operational functions. Clinical service includes drug utilization, providing patients with the proper medication and dosages at the right time for a reasonable cost. Other aspects of clinical service include:

- Drug therapy selection and review screening for allergies, drug/drug interaction and food/drug interactions.
- A pharmacy and therapeutic committee reviews state-of-the-art drug therapy, drug information, formulary service and antidote information.
- An educational program provided to patients and hospital staff, and pharmacy staff development that includes continuing

education, a pharmacy intervention workshop and continuous training and competency assessment.

- Patient assistance programs allowing for free medications for eligible patients through major drug companies and various privately funded programs.

Operational functions include :

- Drug procurement, contracting and purchasing for special drug orders; for example, chemotherapy drugs for cancer patients.
- Drug packaging to decrease waste and ensure convenient administration.
- Unit-dosed drug distribution to prevent error.
- A medication storage-ordering system to provide staff with 24-hour accessability to drugs for emergencies and first-dose medication.
- Drug preparation that includes IV admixture and special compounding.
- Administrative compliance with drug control department
- Planning, organizing and directing policies and procedures in accordance with established policies of the hospital.
- Quality assurance functions that include unit inspections for drug safety, tracking of medication errors and adverse drug reactions and participation in the FDA's Medwatch program.

Objectives of Hospital Pharmacy

The primary purpose of the Hospital of Pharmacy is to care for the patients through the responsible provision of pharmaceutical care. The department is also dedicated to the education of healthcare professionals, conducting research in the pharmaceutical and medical sciences, and to the promotion of public health.

More specifically, the Hospital of Pharmacy seeks to :

- Provide optimal drug therapy for all patients in order to improve their quality of life.
- Provide education and training to pharmacy students, graduate students and pharmacy residents wishing to further expand their experience in pharmacy practice. Such residency training shall meet and exceed the Accreditation Standards approved by the Pharmacy council of India.
- Cooperate with other department in the education of medical, nursing, pharmacy and allied health science students.

- Cooperate in all programs whose objectives are to maintain or upgrade the health of the community.
- Conduct pharmaceutical research of a scientific, clinical or administrative nature with the object of improving pharmaceutical services, patient care and the profession of pharmacy as a whole.
- Provide an environment conducive to professional and personal growth in the field of pharmacy.
- The department is committed to effectively achieving these objectives in an efficient and economically responsible manner.
- Attract a greater number of qualified Pharmacist in hospital practice.

Location and Layout

The in-patient setting of hospital pharmacy is unique in a number of ways. The patients treated by a hospital pharmacist will typically have more complicated conditions than those in an ambulatory setting and be taking multiple medications. A staff pharmacist may have exposure to oncology, intravenous medication therapy (IV meds), neonatal care, nutrition, pain therapy, geriatrics, and much more. Staff pharmacists face a varied set of responsibilities including dispensing medication, making purchasing decisions, monitoring drug therapy, preparing IV medication and overseeing drug administration. The location and layout of a hospital pharmacy will vary greatly between hospitals. Some are "centralized", with all of the pharmacy staff and equipment located in a single area of the hospital, usually on one of the lower floors. Another format is the "de-centralized" pharmacy where there is a main pharmacy in a central location but there are also "mini-pharmacies", called satellites, located throughout the hospital at key patient care units. The layout of the pharmacy will depend on the size, needs, resources, and focus of the hospital.

The out-patient pharmacy should be well furnished to give pleasant look. It should be provided proper facilities for waiting patient. It should display educative or informative posters on health for reading to pass leisure time of waiting. From the out-patient pharmacy department, the visitors should have positive image of pharmacy.

Staff and Facilities requirements

The Hospital Pharmacy consists of various departments depending on set up of the hospital. It has generally dispensing department and medical store in small set up but in a big set up, it has also manufacturing, quality control and clinical pharmacy department.

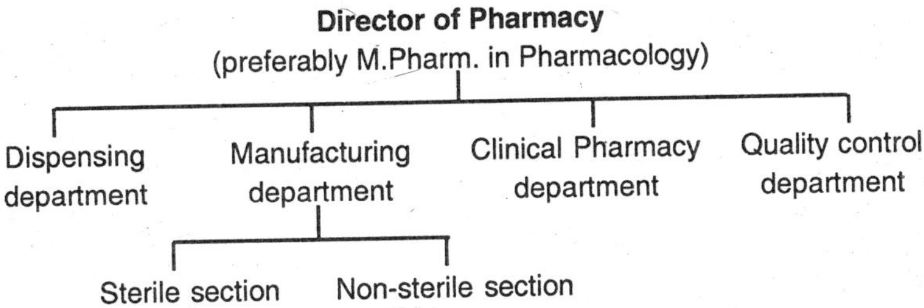

Staff and their qualification

The number of pharmacy staff members depend on:

(i) Number of beds in the hospital
(ii) Scope of service-out-patient and in-patient
(iii) Activities of pharmacy, whether it is involved in manufacturing of drugs and formulations
(iv) Whether the pharmacy stocks and dispenses surgical and laboratory supplies

General directions for number of staff members are as follows :

(i) One Chief Pharmacist or Director of Pharmacy
(ii) One Registered Pharmacist for an average total 60 patient with minimum of 4 pharmacists for smaller hospitals. Total patients include in-patients and out-patients.
(iii) Adequate number of assistant, attendants and safai karamcharies.
(iv) Pharmacist cum clerk, number of which depends on the size of hospital.
(v) If the hospital pharmacy involved in manufacturing of drugs and formulations, it should also have manufacturing chemists and analytial chemists. They should have additional assistant pharmacists.
(vi) For 50 bedded, 100 bedded, 200 bedded, 300 bedded, 500 bedded hospitals, 3, 5, 8, 10, and 15 pharmacists are required. For a big sized hospital, one pharmacist is recommended for 133 patients.

Qualification: The Chief Pharmacist or director should have minimum post graduate degree in pharmacy preferably in hospital pharmacy or pharmacology. Manufacturing chemist should be graduate in Pharmacy with 18 months experience in manufacturing process of drugs and formulations. Analytical chemist should be post graduate in Pharmaceutical Chemistry or Analytical Chemistry. Registered Pharmacist and Pharmacist-cum-Clerk should have Diploma in Pharmacy and should be registered in state pharmacy council.

Equipments required in Hospital Pharmacy

Following is illustrative list of items, needed in a hospital pharmacy department. These may be categorized as :

a) Professional equipments

(i) Balances
(ii) Cabinets (metallic or woood)
(iii) Distilled water manufacturing plant
(iv) Mixing tanks
(v) Filters
(vi) Emulsifiers/homogenisers
(vii) Ointment slab
(viii) Autoclave
(ix) Oven
(x) Pressure pump
(xi) Vacuum pump
(xii) Capsule filling machine
(xiii) Colorimeter
(xiv) Polarimeter
(xv) pH meter
(xvi) Colorimeter

b) Administrative equipments

(i) Book cases
(ii) Notice board
(iii) Computer
(iv) Calculators
(v) Cash register
(vi) Desk
(vii) file cabinets
(viii) Lockers
(ix) Working tables
(x) Camera to monitor the work

From the above lists of equipments, some are fixed and others are movable equipments. Fixed equipments become a part of a permanent part of building and usually include in construction contract, for example, cabinets, counters, sinks and elevators. Movable equipments can be moved from one place to another, for example, balances, mixers and desks.

Floor space

The space requirement of a hospital pharmacy depends on the number of beds, number& types of sub departments and number and types of out-patients. Minimum requirements including space related to manufacture of drug and pharmaceuticals are laid down in Schedule M of drug and cosmetic acts.

The pharmacy requires a minimum of 250 sq feet for any hospital. The floor area recommended for 50, 100 and 200 bedded hospital is as mentioned in Table 3.1. Additional 5 sq. feet per bed is required in big sized hospital. Additional storage space of approximately 170 sq. feet per 100 beds is recommended for bulk storage beneath the Pharmacy.

Table 3.1. Floor Space requirements for Hospital Pharmacies

Department	*Area in sq.ft.*		
	50 beds	*100 beds*	*200 beds*
1. Compounding and dispensing	205	320	495
2. Parenteral	–	185	200
3. Storage	–	125	200
4. Manufacturing	–	–	120
5. Offices and laboratories	–	–	105
6. Circulation	–	–	60

Flow Chart of Patient

There are three steps followed by patients in hospital.

Step I : It is the registration step where the patient is registered and get the card after paying the nominal fees.

Step II : In this general physiological parameters e.g. weight and height, are recorded and guided to respective clinical department on the basis of symptoms reported by the patient.

Step III : In this majority of patients come to pharmacy for medicine and rest of patients are admitted or returned after giving advice. Pharmacy may give the triplicate bill to the patients for deposition of money at the cash counter. After showing the paid receipt, he gets the medicine.

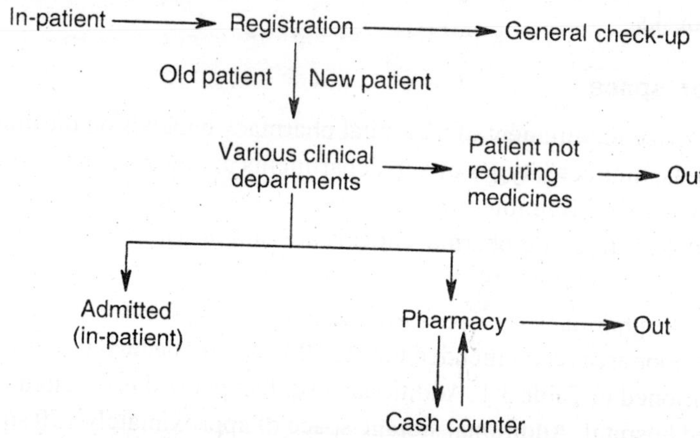

Fig. 3.1. Flow chart of patient in hospitals.

Flow Chat for Pharmaceuticals/Drugs

Pharmacist has both receiving and distribution functions. Pharmacist receives the drugs from main medical stores or sometimes directly from manufacturing units and then distributes to the in-patients and out-patients. Generally quality control tests are performed before entry in pharmacy.

General illustration of flow of pharmaceuticals/drugs is given in Fig 3.2.

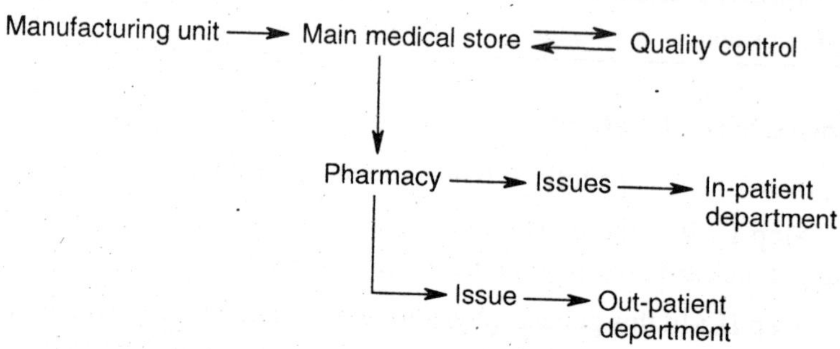

Fig. 3.2. Flow chart of Pharmaceuticals/drugs in hospitals.

Abilities Required by Hospital Pharmacists

The qualified Hospital Pharmacists must have:

1. Knowledge of drugs and their action

Hospital Pharmacist is always associated with the medical staff so he must have knowledge in the medicinal chemistry, pharmacology, route of administration, stability and other information to drugs.

The Hospital Pharmacist must be able to provide information and assistance in the proper handling of drugs.

2. Knowledge of pharmaceutical manufacturing procedure

Usually drugs are required in large quantities in a big sized hospital which may be manufactured in the hospital itself or procured from outside sources. The Hospital Pharmacist must be able to evaluate the relative savings that may be possible by manufacturing drugs in bulk quantities provided cost of labour and maintenance cost are not so much high.

The clinical staff often requests the Pharmacist to prepare drugs in the forms which are not commercially available. Therefore, Hospital Pharmacist must be ready to give this service that generally not expected from him in orher circumstances.

3. Knowledge of quality control procedures

Drugs are purchased or dispensed but in each case, it must be evaluated for its quality and standards laid down in official compendia/ pharmacopoeia. The Hospital Pharmacist must has complete knowledge of Pharmaceutical properties and control procedure to assure a quality product as well as standards prescribed in the official Pharmacopoeia.

4. Participation in research activity

The Hospital Pharmacist must be able to participate or perform research related to improve the usefulness of Pharmaceutical preparation, method of preservation & stabilization and increasing therapeutic effectiveness.

5. Teaching /Training programme

The Hospital Pharmacist must be capable of organizing teaching/ training programme in hospital. He may prepare lectures and demonstration for the nursing staff covering such topics as storage of drugs, drug usage, dosage forms and calculation of dose. Topics such as prescription writing, drug usage and incompatibilities may be presented to the medical staff.

6. Administration and management ability

Under general direction, the chief Hospital Pharmacist has the total responsibility for the direction, management, and administration of all operations of a modern pharmacy in a tertiary care medical center, with special emphasis on program development and implementation. Operations include round the clock in-patient and out-patient dispensaries, the preparation of intravenous and parenteral solutions, in-service education, and inventory control and security. Supervision is exercised over a substantial number of pharmacists and supportive staff. He also stablish operating guidelines for all Pharmacy services in compliance with medical center policies and any other rules and regulations established by regulatory agencies and boards. He also does related work as required. Hence, he should possess the required management and administrative abilities.

4

Chapter

The Pharmacy and Therapeutics Committee

The multiplicity of drugs available and the complexities in the surrounding have made necessary for organized health care settings to have a sound program for maximizing safe, effective and rational drug use. The Pharmacy and Therapeutics (P&T) Committee, or its equivalent, is the organizational keystone to this program.

The P&T Committee evaluates the clinical use of drugs, develops policies for managing drug use and drug administration, and manages the formulary system. This committee is composed of physicians, pharmacists, and other health professionals selected with the guidance of the medical staff. The Pharmacy and Therapeutics (P&T) Committee is an important medical staff advisory group. As the primary, formal communication link between the pharmacy and medical staff, the P&T Committee is of particular importance to the Division of Pharmacy in a hospital.

It is a policy-recommending body to the medical staff and the administration of the organization on matters related to the therapeutic use of drugs.

Objectives

The primary purposes of the P&T Committee are :

1. *Policy Development* : The Committee formulates policies regarding evaluation, selection, and therapeutic use of drugs and related devices.
2. *Education* : The Committee recommends or assists in the formulation of programs designed to meet the needs of the professional staff (physicians, nurses, pharmacists, and other

health-care practitioners) for complete current knowledge on matters related to drugs and drug use.

3. *Advisory* : The P&T Committee is an advisory group of the medical staff. Members of the Committee include representatives from medical staff, pharmacy, nursing, and administration.
   The Committee recommends the addition or deletion of Formulary drugs, monitors and evaluates medication use, and develops and implements policies for appropriate drug use on campus. The members of the P&T Committee look forward to working with you to assure safe and effective drug use at our institution. Questions should be referred to the Chairman of the P&T Committee.
4. *Drug safety* : The Pharmacy and Therapeutics (P&T) Committee conducts in-depth evaluations of available drugs and recommend appropriate drugs for preferred status. For this, drugs/drug classes are evaluated for their safety, efficacy, and overall therapeutics cost value, and then committee makes subsequent recommendations to the Executive Director regarding prior authorization criteria for these drugs and classes

Organization and Operation

While the composition and operation of the P&T Committee might vary among specific practice sites, the following generally apply:

1. The P&T Committee should be composed of at least the following elective members:
   (i) physicians,
   (ii) pharmacists,
   (iii) nurses,
   (iv) administrators,
   (v) quality-assurance coordinators,
   (vi) ex-officio member of committee and others as appropriate.

   The size of the committee may vary depending on the scope of services provided by the organization. Committee members should be appointed by a governing unit or authorized official of the organized medical staff. A chairperson from among the physician representatives is appointed. Generally, a pharmacist is be designated as secretary.
2. They should meet regularly, at least six times per year, and more often when necessary.

3. The committee should invite to its meetings persons within or outside the organization who can contribute specialized or unique knowledge, skills and judgments.
4. An agenda and supplementary materials (including minutes of the previous meeting) should be prepared by the secretary and submitted to committee members in sufficient time before each meeting for them to review the material properly.
5. The minutes of Committee meetings should be prepared by the secretary and maintained in the permanent records of the organisation.
6. Recommendations of the Committee should be presented to the medical staff or its appropriate committee for adoption or recommendation.
7. Liaison with other Organizational Committees concerned with drug use should be maintained.
8. Actions of the Committee should be routinely communicated to the various health care personnel involved in the care of the patient.
9. The committee should be organized and operated in a manner that ensures the objectivity and credibility of its recommendations. The committee should establish a conflict of interest policy with respect to committee recommendations and actions.
10. In formulating drug use policies for the organization, the Committee should be attentive to the content and changes in pertinent guidelines and policies of professional organizations and standards-setting bodies such as the American Society of Hospital Pharmacists, the American Hospital Association, Medical and Nursing Associations, the Joint Commission on Accreditation of Healthcare Organizations, governmental agencies, and others as appropriate.

Functions and Scope

The basic organization of each health care setting and its medical staff may influence the specific functions and scope of the P&T Committee. The following list of committee functions is offered as a guide:

1. To serve in an evaluative, educational, and advisory capacity to the medical staff and organizational administration in all matters pertaining to the use of drugs (including investigational drugs).

2. To develop a formulary of drugs accepted for use in the organisation and provide for its constant revision.
   The selection of items to be included in the formulary should be based on objective evaluation of their relative therapeutic merits, safety, and cost. The Committee should minimize duplication of the same basic drug type, drug entity, or drug product.
3. To establish programs and procedures that help ensure safe and effective drug therapy.
4. To establish programs and procedures that help ensure cost-effective drug therapy.
5. To establish or plan suitable educational programs for the organization's professional staff on matters related to drug use.
6. To participate in quality-assurance activities related to distribution, administration, and use of medications.
7. To monitor and evaluate adverse drug (including, but not limited to, biologics and vaccines) reactions in the health-care setting and to make appropriate recommendations to prevent their occurrence.
8. To initiate or direct (or both) drug use evaluation programs and studies, review the results of such activities, and make appropriate recommendations to optimize drug use.
9. To advise the pharmacy department in the implementation of effective drug distribution and control procedures.
10. To disseminate information on its actions and approved recommendations to all organisational health-care staff.

Role of P&T in Drug Safety

For client safety, P&T Committee designed a system, which checks each new prescription for possible problems before a client receives the medication. The purpose is to prevent a new medication from causing a client more health problems.

When a client takes a prescription to a pharmacist, the pharmacist bills the prescription through the Medicaid computer program. The program checks the prescription against certain drug criteria, and against all other prescriptions that the client has filled through Medicaid. It does not matter where the client filled the prescription. Prescriptions filled at any pharmacy through Medicaid are kept in the computer files.

Here are the criteria the computer checks on prescriptions :

1. Is the dosage of the prescription below the minimum dose or above the maximum dose?
2. Is the prescription a duplicate of another drug given to the client?
3. Will the medication have an interaction with another drug given to the client?
4. Could the medication cause a health problem for client if he or she has certain medical conditions such as diabetes or is pregnant?

The computer program looks for problems which could be very serious, even life threatening. If the program finds a possible problem, the pharmacist sees a warning message. He will share the information with the client, and can contact the prescriber if necessary.

Role of P&T Committe in Emergency Drug List

Each nursing unit or patient care area maintains a standardized emergency box, containing emergency medications to be used in emergency situation. Once the tamper proof lock (for the use) is broken the emergency box should be returned to the pharmacy for the exchange of a complete emergency box. The complete contents of this standardized box is listed in the hospital formulary, recommended by the P&T Committee. Generally, the emergency box contains different syringes, needles, cutters, drugs like aminophylline, amyl nitrite, atropine sulphate, digoxin, saline injection, ringers solution. This list is constantly reviewed by P&T Committee.

Role of P&T Committe in Adverse Drug Reporting

To ensure continued patient drug therapy safety and to fulfill the role of a major medical center in the promotion of good health care, all Adverse Drug Reactions (ADR) must be reported. The Pharmacy and Therapeutics Committee has defined an adverse drug reaction as: any untoward reaction which is associated with drug therapy and meets any of the following criteria :

(i) Requires treatment with prescription medication
(ii) Results in or prolongs patient hospitalization
(iii) Results in permanent or temporary disability
(iv) Results in patient death
(v) Requires reporting to the Food and Drug Administration

These reports may include reactions already listed in the package insert. A causal relationship does not have to be established between the drug and the reaction, it may only be suspected.

If the patient is on multiple drug therapy, the most likely agent or agents should be listed. Any physician, nurse, pharmacist or other health care professional identifying a possible adverse drug reaction can file a report. An ADR report may be filed by telephone or by completing a form.

Forms are kept on all nursing units and in recovery rooms. The time to complete a form is minimal. The patient's address, the name of the reporter and the name of the institution reporting the ADR is held confidential and protected from public disclosure. Completed forms should be given to the pharmacy department by placing them in the pharmacist's order bin on the nursing unit.

Reporters can designate that the reaction should be reported to the FDA by checking the appropriate box. The more detailed FDA reporting form will then be completed by the pharmacy department.

Any questions concerning **Adverse Drug Reaction** reporting should be referred to the Drug Information Center.

Role of P&T Committee in Drug Utilisation

The P&T Committee continuously evaluates prescribing patterns, dispensing and patient drug use with predetermined criteria for the explicit purpose of assessing the safety, effectiveness and appropriateness of drug therapy. An additional component of Drug utilization Review (DUR) is the development and implementation of activities to correct and improve prescribing, dispensing and patient drug use. It may be prospective, retrospective or concurrent.

In every hospital organization, there is preferred drug list (PDL). The PDL is composed of drugs that are medically appropriate and less expensive than other drugs in the same class. The drugs are chosen for inclusion on the list by a Pharmaceutical and Therapeutics Committee (P&T Committee). The P&T membership includes clinicians from various specialty areas and includes public advocates.

All matters pertaining to the use of medications within the institution, including pharmacy programs, must be reviewed and approved through the committee. In addition, medication formulary data is reviewed through the committee and recommendations are offered to the medical staff. Such a wide diversification of involvement and activity necessitates the effective communication between all committee members. An active involvement in the committee by the department of pharmacy services is vital in order to develop a contemporary and progressive institutional pharmacy program. This series of four articles will address several important aspects of the committee's operation, including committee formation, mechanics, operation, and problem solving.

Role of P&T in Drug Product Reporting Program

The drugs purchased/supplied in Hospital may not be of good quality. Any drug product suspected of having a defect should be reported to the drug control department or drug manufacturer for this suspected drug defect.

Role of P&T in Educational Program

The Committee can provide for active and ongoing educational outreach programs to educate providers regarding common therapy problems to improve prescribing and dispensing practices. The Committee shall make recommendations through the educational outreach program via: information dissemination and written, oral or electronic reminders containing patient and/or drug specific information and suggested changes in prescribing or dispensing practices. The Committee may also conduct intensified reviews or monitoring of selected prescribers or pharmacists.

5
Chapter

Drug Distribution System

All Hospital use in large measure, drugs and therapeutic substances, both in-patient and out-patient substances. They are of such a variety that they are hardly understood by the patients most of the time. The bigger the hospital organisation, more the problem of procurement and distribution. There are two types of drug distribution system in Hospitals. Firstly distribution of drugs in in-patient department, operation theatre, radiology department and other specified department. Secondly, drugs are distributed to the patients which donot occupy bed and not admitted, means out-patient department.

(A) DRUG DISTRIBUTION SYSTEM TO INDOOR PATIENTS

Generally, four systems of drug distribution are in use in different hospits in India.

1. Individual Prescription order system

It is a old system but still followed in small private hospitals. In this, doctors write a prescription and ask the patient to get the medication from the licenced retail pharmacy. Sometimes, the information is transcribed by the nurse from the medication order form, prepared by the physician. The pharmacy then dispenses the medication for administration to the patients.

Advantages

(i) Reduction in number of staffs in the hospital

(ii) The prescription is directly reviewed by the qualified pharmacist at the retail pharmacy.

(iii) The system provides the interaction of physician, pharmacists and the patients.

Disadvantages

(i) The retail pharmacy has little patient information and cannot monitor the medication utilization.

(ii) This system is costly because patient has to pay the retail price of medicines.

(iii) Lot of time is lost in procurring of drug from the retail pharmacy.

2. Complete floor stock system

Before the 1960's, medication preparation, distribution, and administration practices had relatively few in-process to checks to ensure that patients received the proper doses of medication as prescribed by the physician. Most healthcare organizations utilized a "floor stock system" where the pharmacist dispensed multiple-dose, bulk supplies of drugs to the patient care area where the nurse then prepared all individual doses of medication intended for administration to the patient. Supplies of medication sent to the patient care unit were not labeled for specific patients and were, therefore, available for several doses for numerous patients. There are two types of drugs :

(a) *'Charge' drugs* : These are costly and obtained from pharmacy stores upon the receipt of prescription/medication order for the individual patient. The cost of drug is billed in the patient account for the charging.

(b) *'Non Charge' drugs* : Generally, these are cheaper and commonly used drugs. The cost of these drugs is not directly in the patient account but included into the day to day cost of hospital ward/ room.

Advantages

(i) Easy and prompt delivery of required drugs

(ii) Elimination of drugs returns

(iii) Reduction in number of staffs required

(iv) Reduction in the number of drug order transcription for the pharmacy.

Disadvantages

(i) The pharmacist did not review the patient's medication order written by the physician, and the doses prepared by the nurse were not checked by anyone else prior to administration. The opportunity for medication errors was substantial. It means, there are greater chances of drug interaction/adverse drug reactions.

(ii) Increased drug delivery on the pavilions

(iii) Adequate space for medication storage in patient care unit is required.

(iv) Potential for drug diversion and misappropriation, resulting in drug loss.

(v) Greater load upon the nurse time.

3. Combination of Individual Drug Order and Floor Stock System

This system is followed in government and also in private hospitals who run on the basis of no profit and no loss. Individual prescription or medication system is followed as a major means. Requirement of drugs/surgical items are given to the patient who purchase and deposit these items in hospital wards/rooms under the supervision of registered nurse. In addition to the above system, limited floor stock system is also used.

Selection of 'Charge' Floor stock Drugs

The decision to which drugs should be placed under the category of 'charge' drugs depends on pharmacy and therapeutic committee (P&TC). Physicians, surgeons and other specialists, who are a members of PTC, have the intimate knowledge of the drugs/other item of the patients within the hospital. Representatives of nursing section, pharmacy and administration should also consulted for guidance/advice.

Once the floor stock list has been finalised, it becomes the duty of hospital pharmacist to enforce the decision of pharmacy and therapeutic committee and make the drug available. The decision of the pharmacy and therapeutic committee should be materialised on priority basis.

Selection of Non-Charge Floor Stock Drugs

A list of non-charge floor stock drugs is prepared on the basis of following criteria :

(i) the cost of preparation

(ii) the frequency of use

(iii) the quantity used

(iv) the hospital budget

(v) reimbursed from third party payers

In India, this list is exceptionally small and, therefore, the patient is billed for numerous single doses of drugs.

A list of pharmaceuticals and related preparations which are considered to be non-charge floor stock drugs, is shown in Table 5.1.

Table 5.1. Pharmaceutical and related preparations

Category	*Preparations*
Anti-allergies	Phenergan injection
	Prednisolone tablet
Antibiotics	Pencillin G potassium injection
	Procaine penicillin injection
Anticoagulant	Heparin 10,000 units/1 ml
Antihypertensive	Reserpine HCl 0.5 mg/2 ml
Cardiovascular agents	Digoxin injection
Diuretics	Frusemide injection B.P.
	Frusemide tablets
Tranquillizers	Chlordiazepoxide 100 mg/2 ml
Miscellaneous	Potassium chloride 49 M Eq/20 ml
	Dextrose 50%
	Manitol injection

Prescribing of Floor Stock Drugs

There are three methods employed in transmitting drug order information from the nursing stations to the pharmacist.

Method 1

Prescription order is written on a separate blank paper by the physician.

Table 4.2. Physician's order form

Physician's order		Name : Regd. No. : Bed No. : Doctor's name :
Date ordered	Date discontinued	Order
4.4.1996		Digitoxin 0.1 mg O.D. in morning
6.4.1996		T. Diazepam 10 mg one H.S.
7.5.1996	8.5.1996	Potassium chloride 1 gm daily in morning

In this method, physician writes the medicine in order form as shown in Table 4.2. Some of the smaller hospital continue to require separate prescription for all medications. There is nothing wrong with this method as it establishes the same professional relationship and follows the same practice which exists in the society.

Method 2

In this method a doctor writes a medicine in order form in duplicate, one copy of which is received by the pharmacist.

Registered nurse or other person posted at nursing station does not need any copy to obtain the prescribed medication as initially ordered.

This system reduces the medication errors because hand written prescription order is directly reviewed by the pharmacist. Physicians are allowed to mix all types of orders for the patients on one sheet. It provides the total picture to the pharmacist what is happening to the patient. It is preferred to educate the physicians to limit the writing of their drug order in a single medication order sheet. Once order is written, it is the duty of other responsible staff members to promptly remove the copy portion and transmit it to the pharmacy in order to avoid dispensing delay.

Method 3

This method is usually adopted in most of the hospitals in India. In this nursing unit incharge transcribes or copies the physician's written order on the another document, sometimes called a drug regulation slip and send it to a pharmacy incharge for reviewing and dispensing. This transcribed or copied order is also used by the pharmacist to create his patient drug profile and to initiate the medication charge.

If the drug is 'non-charge drug', the nurse makes an entry on her records and at the proper time will remove the drug from the ward stock container and administer to the patients.

Labelling of Floor Stock Drugs

It is quite interesting that stock drugs in the ward are not labelled with the direction for use. This is so because number of patients may be receiving the same type of medication but under different therapeutic regimen. If one set of direction is affixed to the container, it may cause confusion and error may result. Therefore, stock medications bear a label which shows the ward number, name and strength of the preparation as well as any other patient information (Fig. 5.1)

Ward No. 3 A
Ibuprofen-Paracetamol Tablet Formula Ibuprofen-400 mg Paracetamol-325 mg

Fig. 5.1. Labelling of floor stock drug.

4. Unit dose dispensing System

In unit-dose dispensing, medication is dispensed in a package that is ready to administer to the patient. It can be used for medications administered by any route, but oral, parenteral, and respiratory routes are especially common. When unit-dose dispensing first began, hospital pharmacies equipped themselves with machines that packaged and labeled tablets and capsules, one pill per package. They also purchased equipment for packaging liquids in unit-doses. As the popularity of this packaging increased, the pharmaceutical industry began prepackaging pills in unit-of-use form. Many hospitals now purchase prepackaged unit-dose medications. However, it is still common for hospital pharmacies to purchase bulk supplies of tablets and capsules from manufacturers and repackage them in the central pharmacy into unit-dose packages. It is important to note that hospitals vary in the proportion of their wards covered by a unit-dose system.

There are many variations of unit-dose dispensing. As just one example, when physicians write orders for inpatients, these orders are sent to the central pharmacy (by pharmacists, nurses, other personnel, or computer). Pharmacists verify these orders and technicians place drugs in unit-dose carts. The carts have drawers in which each patient's medications are placed by pharmacy technicians—one drawer for each patient. The drawers are labeled with the patient's name, ward, room, and bed number. Before the carts are transported to the wards, pharmacists check each drawer's medications for accuracy. Sections of each cart containing all medication drawers for an entire nursing unit often slide out and can be inserted into wheeled medication carts used by nurses during their medication administration cycles. A medication administration recording form sits on top of the cart and is used by the nurse to check-off and initial the time of each administration of each medication. The next day, the carts are retrieved from the wards and replaced by a fresh and updated medication supply. Medications that have been returned to the central pharmacy are credited to the patient's account.

Advantages

(i) Patients receive a letter service and are charged for only doses which are administered to them

(ii) Nurses get more time for patient care as all doses of medication system are prepared in pharmacy.

(iii) Unit dose dispensing allows the pharmacists to check a copy of physician's original order and errors in medication are reduced.

(iv) Paper work is reduced at nursing unit as well as at the pharmacy which saves the time.

(v) Better financial control.

(vi) Pilferage is less

(vii) It prevents the loss of partially used medications

(viii) It does not require storage facilities at the nursing station as in other system.

Disadvantage

Some hospital uses automated machines for unit dose packaging.

The unit dose dispensing concept may be introduced into the hospital in either of two ways :

(a) Centralised Unit Dose Drug distribution system (CUDD).

(b) Decentralised Unit Dose Drug distribution system (DUDD).

The introduction of a unit dose dispensing system in the hospital is not an easy task and requires a planning both within the pharmacy and with in the nursing department. The system should be introduced in a phased manner. He should commence by dispensing injectable in disposable syringes, tablets and capsules in strip-packages, certain lotion, creams and ointment which are already present in unit dosage forms in the market and so lend themselves to the concept of unit dose dispensing.

(a) **Centralised unit dose dispensing :** In this system, all in-patient drugs are dispensed in unit doses and all the drugs are stored in main pharmacy and dispensed at the time, the dose is due to be given to the patient. Drugs are transferred from the pharmacy to the indoor patient by medication carts. Suitable means are required to send a copy of the physician's original medication order to the pharmacy for direct interpretation and filling.

(b) **Decentralised unit dose dispensing :** Small pharmacy often called **Satellite pharmacy** is set up on each floor of the hospital. The main pharmacy procures, manufactures, stores and do the packages of the drug. It supplies the drugs to the satellite pharmacies upon the receipt of medication order. This type of system can be used for a hospital with separate building. General outline of procedure, followed in decentralised unit dose system is mentioned here :

(i) Admission to the hospital, the patient is entered into the system. diagnosis, allergies and other data are entered on patient profile card.

(ii) Medication order copy is sent to the hospital pharmacist.

(iii) Medication order is entered on the patient profile card.

(iv) Pharmacist checks the medication order for allergies, drug-interaction and rationale of therapy.

(v) Dosage scheduled in coordination with the nursing station.

(vi) Medication cart is filled for particular schedule delivery after due inspection.

(vii) Nurse administers the medication and makes appropriate entry on her medication record.

(viii) The medication cart is returned to pharmacy and rechecked.

During the above whole sequence, the pharmacist should be available for consultation by the doctors and nurses.

Emergency Drugs

It consist of life saving medicines like adrenaline, corticorteroids, coramine and insulin. These drugs are placed in a box which is early recognisable and approachable. An emergency box also caries the inventory record of the medicines and its consumption on monthly basis. The hospital pharmacist is responsible for maintenance of emergency medicines.

Bed-side Pharmacy

Hospital pharmacist should be more and more patient oriented. He should work in closed association with nursing and medical staff. Active participation at the ward level by the hospital pharmacist is needed. During his ward visit, a pharmacist should give visit and pass important instruction regarding the drugs to medical/nursing staff. While rendering the services of bed pharmacist, he need not to give up his skill of compounding and dispensing drugs. He should monitor the drugs use by conducting pharmacokinetic studies.

On discharge, the hospital pharmacist should advice regarding the storage and use of medicines.

(B) DRUG DISTRIBUTION SYSTEM IN OUT-PATIENT DEPARTMENT

An out-patient receives general or emergency treatment which could be diagnostic, therapeutic or preventive without being admitted in hospital. An out-patient department is a potent force that keeps a check on patients who need only diagnostic and therapeutic services and not bed. Indoor beds are difficult to establish, maintain and require huge amount of capital. Out-patient department reflects the image of hospital. In India, now-a-days out-patient department is made well organised to attract more and more patient in private hospitals.

Location of Out-patient Pharmacy

It is advantageous to have a separate independent out-patient pharmacy for better service. When it is not practicable specially in small hospital, a combined out-patient and in-patient service can be provided from the same window. Sometimes hospital has combined in-patient and out-patient unit but service is provided from the separate windows.

The out-patients dispensing is done from the same pharmacy where the stock preparations are made together for in-patients and out-patients department. There are two prescription presenting windows - one for men, another for women. The pharmacy receives its supplies from medical stores weekly but emergency supplies can be obtained at any time.

In India, out-patient department and pharmacy are present together in the same building. In some hospitals, they are separated geographically. In such condition, there should be autonomous independent out-patient pharmacy.

Layout of Out-patient Department (OPD)

This document should be well organised for the convenience of patient. It is the department where there is maximum interaction between the public and hospital. The quality of service provided by OPD matters much more.

There should be minimum waiting period for the patients. It can be reduced by providing sufficient space for receiving and filling up prescription.

Waiting rooms should be well furnished with sufficient furniture, reading materials and informative postess. If there is a rush in OPD, more staff members should be provided but it increase the expenses.

Dispensing of Medications in OPD

Patient in his first visit to OPD goes to the registration counter where he is registered himself and guided for medical department on the basis of the clinical symptoms. If the patient is coming by second time, he takes his case file from the registration counter and goes to the respective medical department.

The physician writes the prescription and the patient takes it to the pharmacy where it is dispensed by a pharmacist. If there is a waiting period, the pharmacist gives the token on which basis the patient can be identified. Each prescription is filed properly packaged and labelled. Name, registration number, age, direction if any are provided on the label.

The prescription is recorded in the register. While handling over the dispensed drugs, correct delivery is ensured by checking the token number.

Type of Prescription Received

Depending upon the kind of hospital, the OPD receives the prescription from the following type of patients :

1. General public (generally in Government hospitals or charitable hospitals).
2. Referred patient : These type of patients are referred by primary health centres for diagnosis or further treatment.
3. Patients who have been discharged from the hospital means in-door patients.
4. Private patient : It is a concept of private hospital. There is a

separate time for private patient in which hospital charges consultation fees.

Pricing of Prescriptions

It is necessary to charge from patients for dispensing of prescription in order to meet the expenses of pharmacy. Costing the prescription is a policy matter decided by hospital management in consultation with pharmacy incharge. Low income group patients are exempted from costing or they are charged at concessional rate. Prescription cost can be calculated by adding conversion cost into material cost. Conversion cost is worked out in accordance with an established procedure of costing. It also includes the element of profit, decided in consultation with the management. Material cost includes the cost of main medicament and other pharmaceutical ingredients, e.g., averages and packaging materials.

6

Chapter

Central Supply Services

The central supply department of a hospital is defined as 'centralised department' which provides professioal supplies and other equipments to all specialised departments. This includes both sterile and non-sterile items. Specialised department includes all nursing wards, clinics, laboratories (e.g. pathological, cardiac) and operation theatre.

Central sterile services is restrictive, and it is an old concept in which it supplies the re-usable material only. It has wash room with sterilizing facilities.

Now-a-days central supply services provides the single dose disposable syringes, tubing, urine collection sets, intravenous administration sets, needles, gloves and blood bags. In addition to the above items, it may also involved in cleaning, storage and dispensing of specialised equipments such as suction pumps, cardiac catheters, monitoring equipments, surgical dressing carts as well as preparation of intravenous fluid and surgical irrigating fluid.

Control of Central Supply Services

There are three views regarding the control of central supply services:

1. **Pharmacy control :** In this, central supply services are controlled by pharmacy staff members as they already perform nearly the same duties (procurement, storage and distribution of supplies as well as preparation of various sterile solution) in pharmacy department.
2. **Nursing control :** Majority of items supplied by central supply department are used by nurses for their patients and they are more

familiar with the use of these items. On this basis, central supply services may be kept under the control of nursing department.

3. **Pharmacy and nursing control :** Central supply department has dual function, namely the cleaning, packaging and distribution of medical equipment and supply as well as the manufacture of sterile fluids. First function is controlled by nursing department and second function is controlled by pharmacy department.

Central Supply Department in the Hospitals

Like pharmacy, central supply department has not been granted independent departmental status. It is considered as sub-department under the control of nursing services or surgical services in most of the hospital. Under this type of organisation, incharge of the center supply department does not report to the administrator of hospital or his assistant but to some major departmental head.

In other hospitals, the manufacture of sterile injectable or irrigating solution is separated from the central supply department. This is put separately under the charge of pharmacist. Pharmacy and central supply department share duties. Pharmacist prepares solution, packages the solution for sterilisation, prepares a mixture of chemicals in dry state and then to central supply department for sterilisation and distribution of other specialised department. This method is economical as there is no need to install the sterilising equipment at both the places in pharmacy and central supply departments.

Hospital Pharmacist and Central Sterile Supply

Present pharmacy curriculum in India provides the students sufficient exposure to microbiology, the principles of sterilisation, accounting, computer method and management. Therefore, a pharmacist is educationally better qualified to manage the central sterile supply room in comparison to a nurse. No doubt, nurse has a better knowledge of ultimate use of product supplied. Nursing profession is devoted to the direct care of the patient and, therefore, does not require training in the principle of procurement, packaging, storage and dispensing whereas the pharmacy profession is devoted in providing the various services associated with the needs of doctors, nurses and patients and, therefore, require scientific knowledge.

The pharmacist performs many functions in his daily routine which are either identical or closely resemble to those which are performed by his counterparts in central supply room. These functions are mainly procurement, storage, dispensing, manufacturing in bulks or small lots and teaching and training to various groups.

Close picture shows that pharmacist is better qualified both by education and experience to supervises the central sterile supply services.

Recruitment of Staff in Central Sterile Supply (CSS) Department

Individuals, who are recruited, must be trained about the principles of sterilisation, autoclaving, basic microbiological techniques and biological testings. Most of applicants do not have any prior experience so they must be trained. Job training programme is time consuming, varies from hospital to hospital and is costly to the institution. Therefore, the incharge of CSS department should undertake a technician training programme for qualified person.

Location of Central Sterile Supply Department

Central sterile supply room should be centrally located. It should be situated near to area from which it receives most of the supplies and also from the departments which are its largest consumers.

If central sterile supply department is controlled by the pharmacy department, then these two units should be physically combined or at least adjacent to one another for better supervision by pharmacy personnel.

Central sterile department has a layout as shown in Fig. 5.1. It consists of a series of working stations in 'dirty areas' which are separated from "clean area" by autoclaving and sterilising equipments. The number, type and size of working stations depend on size, nature of hospital, the quantity of disposable materials used, the type of sterilisation required and whether the hospital manufactures sterile intravenous fluid or procures from outside.

Non-sterile items enter from one end of the department, pass through various working stations and are sterilised and finally stored in sterile storage area. From this area, these items are supplied to various departments through clean area.

Such layout minimises the cross flow of nonsterile items with those that are clean or sterile thereby, eliminating the possibility of errors and contamination.

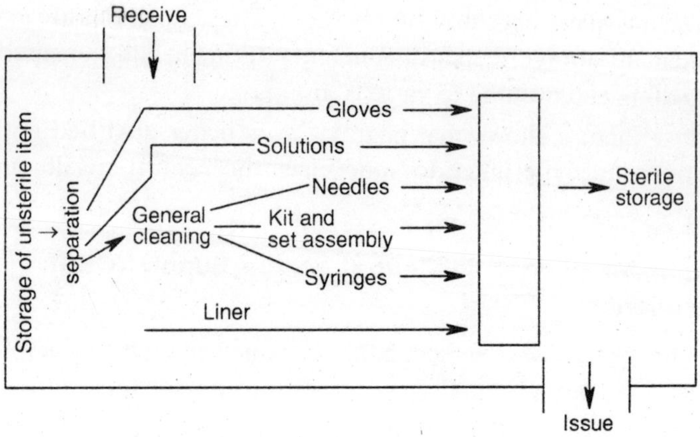

Fig. 5.1. Layout of a central sterile service.

Laminar Air Flow

Laminar air flow is defined as air flow in which the entire body of air within a confined area moves with uniform velocity along parallel flow lines, with a minimum of eddies (Fig. 7.3).

Generally big size hospitals manufacture intravenous fluid, themselves so they must have laminar air flow in central sterile supply department. It provides the microfiltered air over working area and keep away dirt particles from entering in the working area.

The Standardisation Committee

This committee standardises the procedures and equipments used in central sterile supply department. It consists of members from administration, clinical laboratories, department of surgery, medicine, radiology, pathology, nursing, pharmacy and central supply department.

The committee also prepares a standardisation manual or current practice manual.

7
Chapter

Hospital Manufacturing

Economic and Demand Consideration

Hospitals need the large number of items including drugs which may be obtained from market or may be manufactured in the hospital premises. Now-a-days most of the drugs are still procured from outside sources but some hospitals have sterile manufacturing unit to prepare intravenous fluid.

Apart from sterile manufacture, operations are present to prepare non-sterile orals, externals and bulk concentrates. As organisation procures raw material for such manufacturing from market, they must have quality control unit for testing.

The decisions of manufacturing or purchasing the drugs depend on many factors which are as follows :

Quality

If better quality of any drug can be obtained through hospital manufacturing than the same product available in the markets, it is preferred to adopt the first one, provided it is not costlier. If there is no much difference in quality between these two, then quality is not a deciding factor.

Quantity

The items whose order is small, means it is not needed frequently and is always preferred to get from outside. Similarly items, which are required regularly in large quantities, is preferred to manufacture, provided other factors like cost favours it.

Cost

Comparison of costs of items is done, purchased from outside, or manufacture in hospital. The cost of manufacturing item within hospital includes the cost of raw material, production maintenance of manufacturing plants, salaries of staff and others. Low manufacturing cost favours the manufacturing within hospital.

Service

Availability of item is more assured when a hospital manufactures an items than when purchases from outside. Output can be adjusted to some extent according to the need of an item. Assured supply is a valid reason for manufacturing. Unfair means adopted by outside supplies also force to manufacture the items in hospital.

Demand Consideration

The manufacturing of sterile and non-sterile products within hospital is based on the requirement of the hospital in a given period of time. A correct figure of future demand must be observed before the start of any manufacturing unit.

Three methods for estimation of future demand are as follows :

1. Hospital management on the basis of past experience must estimate the quantity of an item that may be required in future.
2. Extension of past history : Future pattern may be extension of past ones. The past consumption pattern of hospital is extended to the future by making a time series and extrapolating it.
3. Casual models : Need is predicted, e.g. demand for an antibiotics is correlated to the number of user patients with infections every month. Generally, regression analysis is done to conclude an estimate.

STERILE MANUFACTURE

It has been estimated that 40% of all drugs administered in hospitals are given in the form of injections and their use is increasing. Part of this increase in parenteral therapy is due to the wider use of Intravenous (IV) fluids. These fluids are finding greater use as the means of administering drugs in addition to fluid replacement, electrolyte balance restoration, supplementary nutrition and total parenteral nutrition

(TPN). A new area of specialisation has been created for hospital pharmacists who can develop the expertise to prepare these solutions and participate in the administration of solutions. The parenteral prescription is becoming increasingly important in hospitals. Considering the increasing demand for the IV fluids, the big sized hospitals have started manufacturing of these fluids within the hospital pharmacy area.

Large and Small Volume Parenterals

Large volume injections intended to be administered by IV infusion commonly are called IV fluids and are included in the group of sterile products referred to as large volume parenterals. These consists of single-dose injections having a volume of 100 ml or more. IV fluids are packaged in containers having a capacity of 100-1000 ml. Minitype infusion containers of 250 ml capacity are available with 50 and 100 ml partial fills for solutions of drugs when used in "piggyback" technique. In addition to IV fluids, this group also includes irrigation solutions and solutions for dialysis. The parenteral preparations other than these volumes less than 100 ml are included in the category of small volume parenterals.

All the parenterals including the ophthalmic preparations have to be necessarily sterilised and they should be free from living microorganisms. Besides these, there should not be any particular matter and any kind of pyrogen present in these products. In the manufacture of the sterilised products, these things are of foremost importance while developing the process of manufacture of parenterals.

General Manufacturing Process

The preparation of a parenteral product may be considered to encompass four general areas as follows :

1. Selection of components, containers and closures.
2. Production facilitics and procedures.
3. Control of quality.
4. Packaging and labelling.

1. Selection of Components, Containers and Closures

Components

Establishment of specifications to ensure the quality of each of the components of an injection is essential. These specifications will be coordinated with the requirement of the specific formulation and will not necessarily be identical for a particular component if used in several different formulations. The most important compopnent is the vehicle. There are wide variety of vehicles which are selected on the basis of solubility and safety reasons.

Water for injection is most commonly used vehicle. It should be free from pyrogen, microbes and particulate matter. It should be free from carbon dioxide, for example, in drugs like barbiturates or free from O_2 in oxygen sensitive drugs.

In addition to water, there are some co-solvents, used with water to increase the stability of the drug or to reduce its hydrolytic degradation. Commonly used water miscible co-solvents are ethyl alcohol, glycerin, propylene glycol and polyethylene glycol. Non-aqueous hydrophobic solvents like fixed oils may be used if the drug has poor solubility or stability in aqueous solvents. Non-aqueous vehicle should be disposable by the body and should be non-irritant to the tissues. Commonly used fixed oils are pea nut, sesame, corn and cotton seed oil. Besides these, there are other substances added to a product to enhance its stability and for other purposes. These include solubilisers, anti-oxidants, chelating agents, buffers, tonicity contributors, anti-bacterial and antifungal agents, hydrolysis inhibitors and antifoaming agents and numerous other substances for specialised purposes. At the same time, these substances must be prevented from adversely affecting the product and should be non-toxic.

Containers and Closures

Containers and closures are in intimate and prolonged contact with the product and may release substance into or remove ingredients from the product. Assessment and selection of containers and closures are necessary for product formulation to ensure that the product retain its purity, potency and quality during intimate contact with the container throughout its self-life. The various materials used for containers are plastics and glasses. Glass is preferred for clarity reasons. Plastics are light weight, less fragile and easy to handle but most of them are not as clear as glass.

Rubber is material of choice for parenteral products. It can permit the entry of hypodermic needle into injection vials and provides for resealing of the vial after the needle is withdrawn. Rubber closure can be properly fixed in place by an aluminium band.

2. Production Facilities and Procedures

Processing of of parenteral products requires area which is clean and free from microbial contamination.

Arrangement of Area

The production area can be considered in terms of five functional areas: the clean-up area, the compounding area, the aseptic area, the quarantine area and the finishing or packaging area. All of these should be designed and constructed for easy cleaning, appropriate environment control, efficient operation and personnel comfort.

Flow plan : In general, the components for a parenteral product flow from the stockroom for released components either to the compounding area as for ingredients of the formula, or to the clean-up area, as for containers and equipments. (Fig. 7.1 shows the process flow and Fig. 7.2 shows flow of materials through production department). After proper processing in these areas, the components flow into the region of the aseptic area for filling of the product in appropriate containers. From these, the product passes into the quarantine area where it is held until all necessary tests have been performed. If the product has to be sterilized in its final container, its passage normally is interrupted after leaving the asceptic area for subjection to the sterilisation process. Once the results from all tests are known and the product

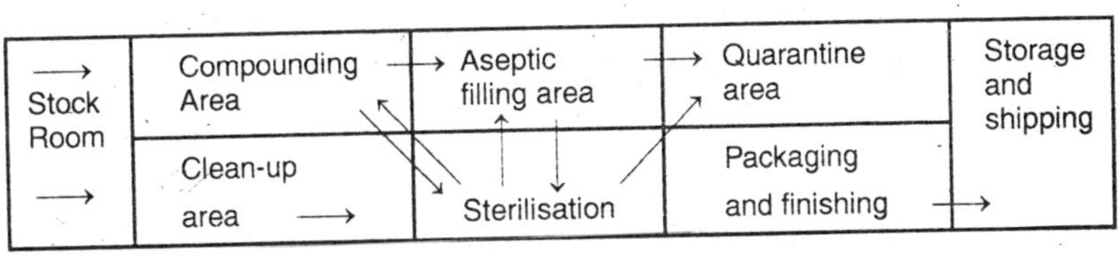

Fig. 7.1. Arrangement of area in sterile manufacturing.

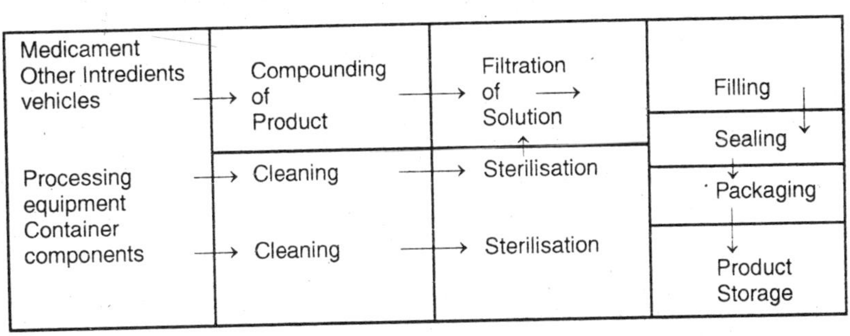

Fig. 7.2. Arrangement of area in sterile manufacturing area.

has been found to comply with its release specifications, it passes to the finishing area for final labelling and packaging. Sometimes there are variations from this flow plan to meet the specific needs of an individual product or to conform to existing facilities.

Aseptic area

This area requires construction features designed for maximum microbial and particulate control. The ceiling walls and floor must be sealed so that they may be washed and sanitised with a disinfectant at needed. All counters should be constructed to stainless steel and attached from the wall so that there are no legs to accumulate dirt where they rest on the floor. All light fixtures, utility service lines and ventilation fixtures should be recessed in walls or ceiling to eliminate ledges joints and other locations for accumulation of dirt and dust. Only product should be fed through hose lines into the area and tanks should be outside. Mechanical equipments should be as completely as possible housed within a stainless steel cabinet.

Personnel

The personnels entering the aseptic area should enter only through an airlock door. They should wear sterile hats, masks, goggles and foot covers. Movement within the room should be minimum and in and out movement rigidly restricted during filling procedure. The requirements for room preparation and personnel may be relaxed some what if the product is to be sterilised terminally in a sealed container. Some are convinced, however, that it is better to have one standard procedure meeting, the most rigid requirements.

The personnels selected to work on the preparation of a parenteral product must be neat, orderly and reliable. They should be in good health and free from dematological conditions that might increase the microbial load. The ill personnels should not be allowed in the aseptic area until their recovery is complete. However, a healthy person with the best of health still sheds some of due viable and non-viable particles from the body. The natural phenomenon creates problems when personals are present in clean rooms, but effective training and proper growing can reduce but not eliminate the problem of particle shedding.

Air Cleaning

The air in these areas can be one of the greatest sources of contamination. So it has to be made free from dust particles as well as micro-organisms. This may be done by a series of treatments that will vary from one installation to the other. In one such series air from onside is first passed through a prefilter, usually of glass wool to remove bigger particles. Then it is passed through an electric precipitator. Such a unit induces an electrostatic charge on particles and remove them by attraction to oppositely charged plates. The air then passed through the most efficient cleaning device, a HEPA (High Efficiency Particulate Air) filter having an efficiency of at least 99.97% in removing particles of 0.3 mm and larger based on the DOP (Dioctyl phathalate) test. Laminar flow of HEPA filtered air is capable of meeting the standard for a class 100 clean room as defined by Federal Standard 209E which states that such an environment contains not more than 10 particles/ft^3 of 0.5 mm and larger size.

The Fig. 7.3 shows a horizontal laminar flow working bench.

Ultraviolet Radiation

Ultraviolet (UV) rays have an antibacterial action, thereby, producing a disinfectant action on directly irradiated surface. Since these rays cannot penetrate a variety of materials, only surface effect is produced. UV rays travel in straight lines only, therefore, objects in the path of light of beam will cast shadows with a resultant lack of irradiation in the shadow area. UV rays are irritating to the skin and particularly the eyes of human beings. Therefore, personnel working irradiation area

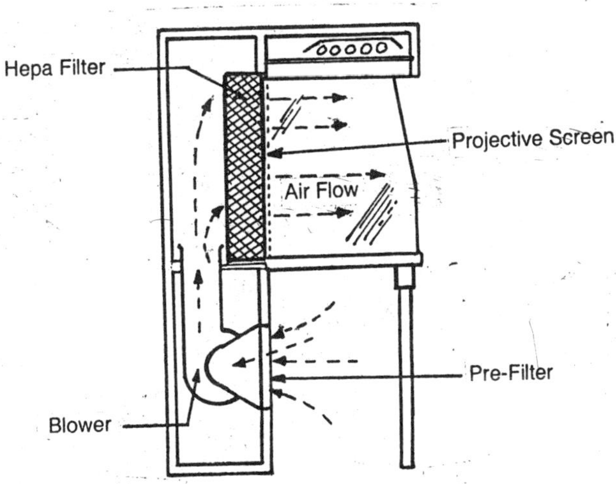

Fig. 7.3. Horizontal laminar flow.

must be protected from direct exposure. The best practical source of UV rays is the cold cathode mercury vapour lamp. This lamp emits a high proportion of radiation at 253.7 mm wavelength. It is generally stated that an irradiation intensity of 20 μw/cm^2 is required for effective antibacterial activity.

Environmental Control Evaluation

Manufacturers of sterile propucts use extensive means of controlling the environment so that these critical products can be prepared free from contamination. Suitable tests should be performed to determine the level of control actually achieved. Normally the tests consist of counting viable and non-viable particles suspended in the air or settled on surfaces in the work space. The tests used generally measure either the particles in a vapour of sampled air or the particles that aresetting or are present on surfaces. A volume of air measured by an electronic particle counter will detect all particles but not differentiate between viable and non-viable ones. However, because of the need to control the level of microbes in the environment in which sterile products are processed, it is also necessary to detect viable particles. These usually are less in number and are only detectable as colony forming units (CFUs) after a suitable incubation period in culture media, for example 30°-35°C for up to 48 hours. To measure the total particle count in air, electronic counters, like counter, are available. Several air sampling devices are used to obtain a count of microbes in a measured volume of air. A widely used method for microbiological sampling consists of exposure of nutrient agar culture plates to the settling of microbes from the air.

Procedure : Mixing, clarification, filling, sealing and sterilisation are the common steps involved in the preparation of parenteral products.

(i) Mixing and clarification

Ingredients are mixed in the mixing tanks or containers. These containers should be free from pyrogens and microbes. Clarification may be achieved by passing the solution under differential pressure through filters, e.g. sintered glass filters, asbestos pad filter, kiselghur filters and membrane filters. The filters must be able to remove as small as approximately 0.2 m. Membrane filter is disposable, efficient and effective. They are inert and have no adverse effect on solution passed through them. Sintered glass and asbestos filters are available in the form of disc whereas unglazed porcelain and kieselghur filters are available in the form of disc as well as candles.

(ii) Filling

The above product is filled in a container under aseptic condition. It consists of transfer of measured quantity from a bulk container to a unit container. Solution sterilized by filtration are to be filled under aseptic conditions.

Initially liquids were filled by using hypodermic needles, burettes and flask but now these are replaced by automatic filling machines which measure the liquid of volume and forced into unit container.

Solids like antibiotics are divided by weighing and then filled into individual containers. Large scale filling device consists of measurement and transfer of a volume of granular material caliberated in terms of weight desired.

For transfer of viscous liquids, a sliding piston valve is used.

(iii) Sealing

Filled container should be sealed as soon as possible to prevent the contents from being contaminated. Ampoule are sealed by melting an upper tip portion of the glass with a fine jet of flame. For rapid sealing, a high temperature gas oxygen flame is most useful.

Vials and bottles are sealed by closing the opening with rubber or plastic closure which is held in position by aluminium caps.

(iv) Sterilisation

It is a process of final removal or destruction of micro-organisms. Parenteral products are generally sterilized after filling and sealing except for thermolabile medicament. This is called terminal sterilisation. Thermostable medicaments are generally sterilized by hot air oven (dry heat method). Other parenteral products are sterilized by autoclaving (moist heat method) which employs steam under pressure.

Thermolabile medicament can be sterilized by filtration through bacteria proof filters during filling under aseptic condition. Other thermolabile products like colloids, emulsion and suspension may require a process of sterilizing each ingredient separately and then product is formulated under aseptic conditions. Sterilization by radiation can also be used for thermolabile medicament, for example penicillin, streptomycin, vitamins and hormonal products are sterilized by ionizing radiation. Gaseous sterilization is also non-thermal method but can not be used as gas can't penetrate the glass or other imperious material to reach the medicament.

3. Control of Quality

Parenteral products are subjected to quality control tests like sterility test, pyrogen test, clarity test and leaker testing before use.

Sterility Test

Sterility test is performed to confirm the absence of micro-organisms.

After random sampling, a suitable amount of parenteral product under test is transferred aseptically into sterile nutrient media and incubated for suitable period at appropriate temperature. After incubation, the presence or absence of microbes is observed by its growth, microbial growth is seen if they are present. The entire test is carried out under aseptic condition. Suitable control tests are also performed in a similar way to check the sterility of test media as well as its ability to support microbial growth. If the parenteral product is itself antimicrobial or contain any bactericidal agent, then it is either diluted or some antagonistic substance is added to prevent the antimicrobial action. For example, if a product contains phenol as bactericidal so it must be diluted so that it becomes ineffective; in the similar way to the penicillin can be counteracted by pencillinase and sulpha drugs can be antagonised by adding para-aminobenzoic acid.

Pyrogen Testing

Pyrogens are lipopolysaccharides in nature. It is metabolic product of microbes and cause pyretic reaction if injected in the body. Pyretic reactions are characterised by fever and chills. Due to this reason, parenteral products are tested for absence of pyrogens.

Pyrogens are tested by injecting parenteral product into sensitive animals like rabbit. The rise in body temperature is observed. The sample passes the pyrogen test if no rabbit shows a rise in body temperature more than 0.6° following injection or sum of the rise for three rabbits exceeds 1.4°C. The pyrogen test should preferably run separately on the vehicle as well as the product under test.

An alternative method called litmus test is used for determination of pyrogenic endotoxins. In this product solution is combined with a cell lysate from blood cells of horseshoe crabe. An endotoxin, if present, will be coagulated with protein fraction of the amoebocytes and cause the gel formation. This test is comparatively simple and more sensitive.

Clarity Testing

Clarity test is performed to observe the presence or absence of a particulate matter. Generally, it is checked by direct lighting on the container against a black and white background. However, this method has its own limitation. The alternative method consists of filtration followed by detection of particles on filter paper under microscope.

Now-a-days automatic image analysis device is used in which image of the particles is focussed on screen. Some methods use the light absorption, light scattering or change in electrical resistance to detect the particular matter.

Leaker Testing

Leaker testing is done to check the leakage of products from ampoules. The sealed containers are dipped into coloured solution generally 1% methylene blue and negative pressure are applied. Under this pressure, there will be an entry of coloured solution if proper sealing is not done. The alternative method consists of autoclaving of the ampoules in a dye bath.

This test is further modified. The hot ampoules from the autoclave is immediately immersed in cold dye solution. Entry of coloured solution into ampoule indicates the improper sealing and should be discarded.

4. Packaging and Labelling

Parenteral products are packed either in single dose containers or in multiple dose containers.

Single dose containers, commonly called ampoules, are sealed by fusion of glass container under aseptic condition. The glass container is made to have a neck portion that may be easily separated from the body of the container without fragmentation of the glass ampoule.

Multiple dose containers are affixed with rubber or plastic closures to permit the penetration of a hypodermic needle without the removal or destruction of the closure.

Parenteral product must be labelled to indicate : (i) name of preparation, (ii) % content of drugs or the amount of drug present in a specified volume or for a drug preparation, the amount of active ingredient present and the volume of liquid to be added to the dry preparation, (iii) route of administration, (iv) a statement of storage condition and an expiry date, (v) name of manufacturer, and (vi) batch number. Preparation intended to be used as dialysis, or irrigation solution should meet the requirement for injection except a label indicating that the solution is not intended to be injected. All containers appropriately labelled should allow a sufficient area of the container to remain free of label for its full length of circumference to permit inspection of the contents.

NON-STERILE MANUFACTURE

The products which present the greatest difficulties in terms of microbial growth are the aqueous systems. During the manufacture and filling of such products, sources of microbial contamination are numerous.

Solution

A solution is a liquid preparation that contains one or more soluble chemical substances dissolved in water. The solute is usually non-volatile. Specific methods of preparation are given in the compendia for most of the solutions. These procedures fall into three main categories :

1. *Simple solutions* : They are prepared by dissolving the solute in a suitable solvent. The solvent may contain the other ingredients which stabilize or solubilize the active ingredient.
2. *Solution by chemical reaction* : They are prepared by reacting two or more solutes with each other in a suitable solvent.
3. *Solution by extraction* : Drugs for pharmaceutical necessities of vegetable or animal origin are often extracted with water or hydro-alcoholic solution.

Equipments : In the most general terms, the equipments used in the manufacture of oral solutions consist of mixing tanks equipped with a mean of agitation, measuring devices for large and small volume of liquids and solids, and a filtration system for the final polishing and/or sterilization of solution. In addition most production facilities are equipped with systems for bulk material handling/discharging equipments. All equipments must be thoroughly cleaned and sanitized before use. Equipments and pipe lines can be sterilized by alcohol, boiling water, autoclaving or dry heat. Tanks are constructed of polished stainless steel and are usually jacketed to allow for heating or cooling of the contents, equipped with see through charging ports and illumination for easy observation of contents. If tanks are used for compounding of the bulk liquid, they have a built-in agitation system. The liquid is then clarified by cycling through a filtration system and the polished solution is stored in an adjacent tank and filling line should be held to a minimum to reduce the microbial contamination. Operators must used head coverings and face masks. Use of portable laminar flow units can be an aid in certain operations.

Emulsions

The preparation of an emulsion requires work to reduce the internal phase into small droplets and disperse them through the external phase. This may be accomplished by a mortar and a pestle or a high speed emulsifier. The addition of emulsifier not only reduces this work but also stabilizes the final emulsion. Emulsion may be prepared by four principle methods.

1. Addition of internal phase to external phase.
2. Addition of external phase to internal phase.
3. Mixing both phases after warming each.
4. Alternate addition of the two phases to the emulsifying agent.

Equipments : In small scale production, the most commonly used equipment is a pestle and a mortal. On a large scale the following equipments used are :

Agitators : Ordinary agitation or shaking may be used to prepare the emulsion. This method is frequently employed by the pharmacist, particularly in the emulsification of easily dispersed low viscosity oils. The mortar and pestle are widely used by the prescription pharmacists in extemporaneous preparation of emulsions, but they can not be used to prepare an emulsion if the emulsifying agent lacks viscosity. Small electric mixers can be used to prepare emulsions at the prescription counter. However, they can't be used if gelatin is an emulsifying agent. Production-size agitators include high powered propeller shaft stirers immersed in a tank or self-contained units with propeller and paddle systems.

Colloid mills : The principle of operation of these is the passage of mixed phases of an emulsion formula between a stator and a high speed roter revolving at speeds of 2000-18000 rpm (Fig. 7.4).

Homogenizers : In these the mixed phases are passed between a finely ground value and seat under high pressure. This in effect produces an atomization which is enhanced by the impact received by the

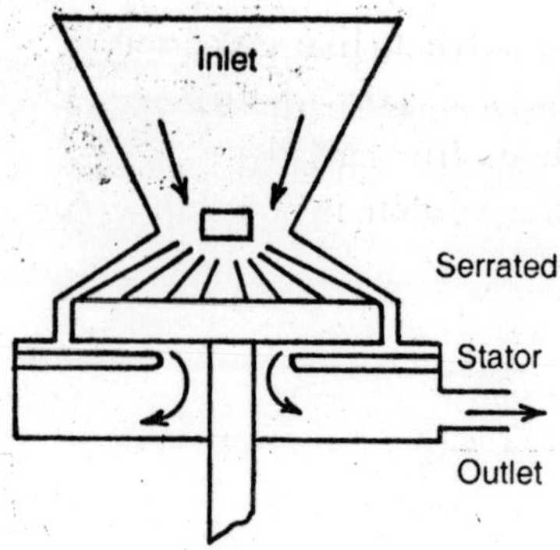

Fig. 7.4. Colloid mill.

automized mixture as it strikes the valve head. For small scale preparation of emulsions, the hand homogenisers are available.

Ultrasonic devices : An oscillator of high frequency (100000-500000/sec) is connected to two electrodes between which is placed a perizoelectric quartz plate. The quartz plate and electrodes are immersed in an oil both and when the oscillator is operating at high frequency, waves flow through the medium.

Emulsification is accomplished by simply immersing a tube containing the emulsion ingredients into this oil bath.

Suspension

The suspensions may be prepared by two methods : (i) Precipitation methods, (ii) Dispersion methods.

Precipitation methods : The substance to be suspended is first obtained in solution form, then it is made to precipitate in a very fine particle size form. It can be accomplished by changing the pH, organic solvent precipitation or double decomposition, etc. If the suspension is made by a dispersion technique, the vehicle must be formulated so that the solid phase is easily wetted and dispersed. A number of dispersion methods are used to prepare suspensions. Milling is the term given to the mechanical process of reducing the particle size which may be accomplished by a number of different types of machines like the hammer mill, ball mill, fluid energy mill and roller mill.

Suspension equipment such as colloid mill or homogenizer normally are used in wet-milling finished suspensions to reduce agglomerates and to form a suitable preparation on a small scale in a pharmacy. The particles should be wetted thoroughly with a small quantity of water miscible solvent, like glycerine or alcohol which reduces the liquid air interfacial tension. Alternatively, a dry suspending agent can be triturated with the drug particles using a small quantity of glycerine or alcohol and then volume is made up with water.

Extracts

They are defined as concentrated preparations of vegetable and animal drugs obtained by removal of active constituents of drugs with menstrum. Evaporation of all or nearly all of the solvent and adjustment of the residual masses or powders to the prescribed standards gives the extracts. Three forms of extracts are recognised : (i) semisolid or liquids of syrupy consistency, (ii) plastic masses, and (iii) dry powders. The extracts are mostly prepared by extracting the drugs by percolation. The percolate is concentrated, generally by distillation under reduced pressure. The other methods of preparing extracts are maceration, digestion, infusion and decoction.

Semi Solids

Irrespective of the method employed for the preparation, semisolids should be smooth and free from granular or gritty particles. In manufacturing, certain general considerations are observed. If insoluble substances are to be incorporated in the semisolid base, they should be impulsable powder form. For efficient incorporation of insoluble substances, they should first be levigated with a small quality and then mixed with the bulk. Water soluble substances are incorporated by first dissolving in small quantity of water and then incorporating it in base. Soluble drug may also be added by fusion method. Remaining substances are then added and mixed by stirring.

Ointment preparation by mechanical incorporation may be achieved by :

1. *Mortar and pestle method* : This method is used to a limited extent in compounding practice particularly when large quantities of liquids are to be incorporated into the base or when base is exceptionally large in quantity.
2. *Ointment slab* : Powder is first rubbed with small quantity of base and then diluted with rest of the base.
3. *Ointment mills* : Most popular ointment mill is the triple roller mill in which ointment is made to pass through narrow clearance between the rollers (Fig. 7.5).

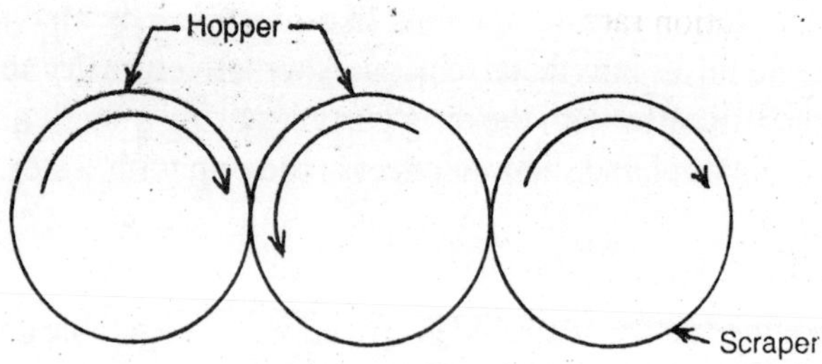

Fig. 7.5. Ointment mill.

The various types of equipments required for manufacturing of non-sterile ointments are mixing and storage tanks, kettle with steam, gas or electrically heated water still or deionizer, colloidal mill or other suitable emulsifier, triple roller mill or ointment mill, vacuum or gravity filters, filter press, liquid fitting equipment, jar or tube filling equipments and filling machines.

Tablets

The various ingredients used in tablet preparation include diluents, binders, lubriants, glidants, disintegrants, colouring agents, flavouring agents, etc. These are basically three sections in a table manufacturing unit.

(a) *Granulating section* : Various powders are mixed with the help of powder mixers and mass mixers and granulated with the help of granulator. After sifting they are dried in ovens.

(b) *Tableting sections* : Absolutely granules dry are compressed into tablets after addition of glidents and lubricants at the time of compression. Various types of tableting machines are used like simple punch, double punch or rotary tableting machine, high speed rotary machines and multilayer rotary tablet machine. Compressed tablets are then taken to the coating section.

(c) *Coating section* : Various kinds of coatings like sugar coating, enteric coating etc. are applied. The equipments used in this section are : jacketed kettle steam, gas of electrically heated, coating pans, polishing pans and heater and exhaust systems.

Besides compressed tablets moulded tablets are also prepared. They are prepared either by hand or hand moulding tablet triturates, or by machine molding and sometimes by compression also. Finally, they are tested for hardness, dimensions, weight variations, disintegration time and dissolution rate.

Quality Control of Raw Materials, Procurement from Stores

Quality control of the finished product is the organised effort of company. The desired features, properties, characteristic, identification, purity, uniformity, potency and stability are maintained within establishment limits. The quality of dosage form should not only be tested at the end but must be built into the product right from the moment of receipt of raw materials through their processing until the final packaging. The four means, namely men, materials, machines and methods mainly, contribute for quality. The quality control through raw materials can be controlled by :

(a) establishment of suitable specifications,
(b) development of adequate test procedures,
(c) specific identification markings,
(d) proper storage conditions,
(e) adequate sampling,
(f) appropriate testing,
(g) requiring compliance with specifications, and
(h) maintenance of records and samples.

The equipments used in the manufacture of products and the conditions in which the processing is done are important for quality product. Building for manufacturing, testing and storage operations are of adequate design, size and should be constructed to :

(a) provide for proper receipt and storage of raw materials,
(b) allow proper segregation and identification of material during manufacturing and packaging,
(c) provide suitable sampling facilities,
(d) provide easiness in maintaining cleanliness and for avoiding contamination,
(e) provide adequate laboratory equipments, and
(f) provide proper storage for final products.

The equipment used in the manufacturing process should be :

1. property located and maintained,
2. constructed to facilitate easy cleaning,
3. non-reactive, non-adsorbent and non-additive, and
4. adequate for the required operations.

Quality Control of Raw Materials Testing

Raw material specifications must be written in precise terminology, must be complete, must provide specific details of test methods, type of instruments and method of sampling and must be properly identified. The following is the list of general tests, limits and other physical and chemical tests for raw materials.

A. *Nomenclature* : It includes the name of the drug, structural formula, molecular weight and the chemical name as prescribed in official compendia.

B. Sample size and sample containers are to be checked.

C. The materials are analysed to assure quality, strength and purity. It includes the assay of the material by a suitable quantitative method of analysis.

D. *Specifications* : This includes description of materials by the use of a number of methods like specific chemical tests, infrared absorption, ultraviolet absorption, melting point, congealing point, boiling point and thin layer, paper, liquid or gas chromatography methods.

E. Purity and quality are checked in a number of ways by physical, chemical and biological methods. In these analyses solubility, pH, ash values, specific rotation, loss on drying, water content, tests for heavy metals, acid value, iodine valve and saponification valve, etc. are carried out. Physical tests useful in formulation include particle size, crystal characteristics and polymorphic forms. Assay of the materials is carried out to assess the purity of the materials. Microbial contamination is checked by certain microbiological tests which are required to be within certain limits prescribed for them.

Procurement of Raw Materials

The pharmacist may be the actual buyer in a small hospital. The main function of pharmacist in purchasing is to establish standards and specifications for all drugs. The use of competitive bidding is considered good practice where a drug is used in large amounts or required in continuity. A quotation request is directed to appropriate manufacturers and the companies with the lowest price and yet with standard quality usually receives the order for the material. After which purchase order is prepared. The materials can be purchased by direct purchase from the manufacturers, from a wholesaler, from a retail pharmacy most likely in emergency or by a contract purchase arrangement with a manufacturer. Contract purchase arrangement may be done by bid from either a manufacturer. Contract purchase arrangement may be done by bid from either a manufacturer or a wholesaler. It is the pharmacist who plays the key role in these procedures. He selects the mode of purchasing. He maintains the list of the names, addresses and telephone numbers of drug manufacturers, wholesalers and local representatives. Pharmacist prepared detailed specification for drugs, chemicals and biologicals.

There are two systems of procurement of drugs in a hospital :

1. *Centralised system* : All the items including drugs are purchased by purchase officer or purchase committee.
2. *Decentralised system* : Purchasing is done by the user department. In this system, pharmacist should purchase or should be consulted as in procurement of drugs as he has responsibility to compound, dispense, manufacture and distribute the drugs in the hospitals.

Procurement Procedure

It consists of following steps :

1. *Purchase requisition* : First of all purchase requisition form is filled for the desired drugs. It consists of data concerning the description, specification, packaging, price, quantity, needed as well as information concerning the inventory balance and anticipated monthly uses. The original of this form is forwarded to administrative officer for approval. Once approved, it is sent to purchase officer while retaining its duplicate copy.
2. *Purchase order* : After the receipt of the purchase requisition, purchase officer prepares a purchase order in a printed form. The items are alphabetically arranged or supplierwise indicating the specification, prices and quantities ordered. Purchase order is prepared in several copies to deliver to the : (i) supplier, (ii) account section, (iii) purchase section, (iv) initiating department from which purchase requisition originated, and (v) receiving section which receive items.

   The purchase order is sent to the supplier.
3. *Receipt of order* : When items arrive in the receiving section, the specification, quantities and prices are checked against the purchase order. If a part of the order is returned to the supplier and the other copy to the concerned department. Against returns, a credit note may be obtained from the supplier.

The items received and entered in the purchase record register having the columns for receipt as well as issues to complete picture of inventory.

Control on Purchases

A proper A, B, C analysis in terms of A, B and C items can be made by estimating the cost of individual items with total amount of purchase order. Items having more cost need better control as compared to low cost items.

A more reliable method is the computation of inventory turnover. Inventory turnover is calculated by dividing the cost of items sold during a financial period by the average of opening and closing inventories.

It gives the number of times the inventory has been 'turned' during the financial period. A low turnover indicates duplication of stock, excess purchase of less running items and dead inventory. High turnover of inventory may be due to small volume purchasing which indicates a failure to take a benefit of the maximum quantity discounts.

A turnover of four times a year is satisfactory for most of the hospitals.

Hospital pharmacists should control the purchasing of items by use of Economic Order Quantity (EOQ) and Recorder Quantity Level (RQL).

The RQL is the inventory level that must be reached before order of same items can be placed. Ideally, the remaining inventory should be depleted before the arrival of new shipment but zero stock level must be avoided as it can cause serious problems.

The determination of how much to order is EOQ factor. In determining EOQ factor, it is important to know the cost of ordering and the cost of carrying inventory. The cost of carrying inventory include the interest cost, storage charges, insurance cost, taxes, obsolescence costs, pilferage/determination/expiry costs.

Dividing th value of the inventory by the total of above costs results in the inventory carrying cost. It is advantageous to order expensive items monthly and cheap items annually. The economic order quantity can be calculated by following formula :

$$\text{EOÇ} = \sqrt{\frac{2 \times 12 \times \text{monthly usage} \times \text{order cost}}{\text{unit cost} \times \text{holding cost}}}$$

8
Chapter

Hospital Formulary System

Today, there is multiplicity of drugs. Out of several brands of medicine, some medicine available in market today are either duplicate or of doubtful value. The care of patients in hospital and other health care facilities very often depends on the effective use of drugs. This enforces the need of complex screening methods for selection of drugs for use within the health care set-up like hospitals.

The basic principle of selection is to provide efficacious and cost effective drugs. The use of appropriate drugs in the hospital can be promoted through the concept of **hospital drug formulary system**. It is an ongoing process whereby a healthcare organization, through its physicians, pharmacists, and other healthcare professionals, establishes policies on the use of drug products and therapies, and identities drug products and therapies that are the most medically appropriate and cost-effective to best serve the health interests of a given patient population. Though the concept of hospital formulary is in practice in the USA and other developed countries, it is yet to gain popularity in Third World countries including India. Chile was the first followed by Sri Lanka were the initial countries to introduce the concept of formulary in the developing world.

Hospital drug formulary is a continually revised compilation of drugs containing important information that reflects the current judgement of medical staff of the hospital. The system consists of maintaining an updated and user-friendly formulary. It is the backbone of drug management process in the hospital.

The development of formulary and its maintenance provide several advantages :–

(i) Promotes rational drug use n Improves healthcare outcomes.
(ii) Improves efficiency in procurement and inventory management.
(iii) Ensures regular supply and availability of essential drugs.
(iv) Decreases significantly the average health care cost.

Development of Hospital formulary

The development of hospital formulary and its management is usually the responsibility of hospital administration through Pharmacy and therapeutic committee or other equivalent body of the hospital. The selection of drugs for use in the hospital is the first requirement of developing a hospital formulary. The selection process is usually based on prevalent disease conditions being treated and the appropriate first choice of treatment for each disease condition as identified using standard treatment guidelines, either nationally or locally developed.

The selection needs to be evidence based on efficacy, safety, quality and cost. The hospitals must have clear guidelines or procedures for adding and deleting drugs from the list for use in the hospital, normally called Essential Drug List or Formulary List.

1. The formulary is a listing of drugs, dosage forms, package sizes, and drug strengths stocked by the hospital. It is published as a quick reference to assist the physician and nursing staffs.
   The contents of formulary are divided into four general sections: the Introduction, a Therapeutic Index, the Drug Monographs, and a General Reference Section.
2. The Therapeutic Index is a listing by pharmacological or therapeutic category of those drugs which are carried in one or more dosage forms, by the pharmacy. The listing is alphabetical by generic name under each category. From the Therapeutic Index, the physician can determine if the desired drug is stocked in any form. If it is, she/he will then refer to the Drug Monographs Section for complete information.
3. The Drug Monographs Section is a straight alphabetical listing of both trade names and generic names. The trade name will be cross referenced to the generic name under which the complete information will be found. Each Complete monograph will contain the following information:
   (a) Official, non-proprietary, or generic name.
   (b) Trade name: Common trade or proprietary names which refer

to the generic drug. The listing of a trade name does not necessarily mean that it is stocked as such by the Pharmacy.

(c) Category: It relates to the information in the Therapeutic Section of the Formulary.

(d) Dosage Form: This lists all the dosage forms which are available in the pharmacy.

(e) **Note:** Information of special interest or of an unusual nature is indicated here. However, the absence of a cautionary note does not necessarily imply that a particular drug may be used without the necessary precaution or discretion.

4. The General Reference Section contains information and aids that are used in patient care. It contains dosing formula conversion tables for weight, measures and temperature, as well as guidelines for use of certain drugs as adopted by the Pharmacy and Therapeutic Committee.
5. Drug items are listed generically in the formulary. Orders for drugs written by hospital physicians are interpreted and filled using generic names.
6. The heart of the formulary system is the Pharmacy & Therapeutics Committee. The Committee is established by the Hospital Medical Board. Membership will be comprised of representatives of the professional departments/services, house staff, nursing, pharmacy, administration.
7. The Committee shall be responsible for the development and surveillance of all drug utilization policies and practices within the hospital in order to assure optimum clinical results and a minimum potential for hazard. The Committee shall assist in the formulation of broad professional policies regarding the evaluation, appraisal, selection, procurement, storage, distribution, use, safety procedures and all other matters relating to drugs in the hospital. It shall perform the following specific functions.

   (a) Serve as an advisory group to the hospital medical staff and the pharmacy on matters pertaining to the choice of available drugs.

   (b) Make recommendations concerning drugs to be stocked on the nursing unit floors and by other services.

   (c) Develop and review the formulary or drug list for use in the hospital.

(d) Prevent unnecessary duplication in stocking drugs and drugs in combination having identical amounts of the same therapeutic ingredients.

(e) Develop and review procedures to control the use of dangerous and toxic drugs with such procedure to be approved by the medical staff.

(f) Develop a procedure for handling and control of drugs brought into the hospital by patients.

(g) Evaluate clinical data concerning new drugs or preparations requested for use in the hospital.

(h) Establish standards concerning the use and control of drugs.

(i) Review of the appropriateness of the empiric and therapeutic use of drugs through the analysis of individual or aggregate patterns of drug practice.

(j) Development of policies and procedures relating to the selection, distribution, handling, use and administration of drugs and diagnostic testing materials.

(k) Review of all significant adverse drug reactions.

8. Additions to the Formulary are made by submitting a "Physician's Request for Addition to the Formulary" to the Secretary of the P&T Committee. Blank Forms can be obtained from the Inpatient Pharmacy. Forms will be forwarded to the physician only.
9. Physicians requesting drug additions to the Hospital Formulary have to review drug usage data on formulary items which are comparable to the agent being requested. Usage data is available from the Pharmacy upon request. The requestor has to assert whether the requested item has a greater therapeutic or economic value than items that are currently available.
10. The Pharmacy Committee meets monthly on the fourth Monday of the month. Requests received within 10 calendar days of the meeting would generally be included on the meeting agenda.
11. *Non-formulary Drugs* : When a non-formulary drug is prescribed, a pharmacist contacts and informs the prescribing physician that the drug is non-formulary and not stocked in the pharmacy. The pharmacist informs the physician of other formulary alternatives available. If the physician feels that the non-formulary drug is still needed, authorization from the attending physician on that

service must be obtained. The housestaff physician contacts the attending physician, who authorizes use of the non-formulary drug by issuing a medication order. If the attending physician determines that the non-formulary drug is needed, the physician should issue a medication order stating such, enter the order in SCM or call the pharmacist to give a verbal order. The drug will then be obtained by pharmacy for a specific patient.

Non-formulary drugs are normally obtained within 24 hours, or as soon as possible from a local wholesaler, community pharmacy, or neighboring hospital.

Principles of Formulary System Management

The purpose for ongoing management of the formulary system is to optimize patient care through rational selection and use of drugs and drug products within the health-care setting.

Pharmacists play a primary role in assessing the relative safety and efficacy of pharmaceuticals nominated for addition to or deletion from the formulary. Through the application of techniques of formulary system management and through reevaluation and improvement of these techniques as necessary, the effectiveness of the formulary system is continuously assessed, resulting in quality improvement of the overall drug use process. Both therapeutic outcomes and costs related to the drug use process can thus be optimized.

Prescriber acceptance of the formulary management process is essential to effect quality improvements through formulary system management. Pharmacists play a key leadership role in fostering this acceptance by clarifying and supporting the goals and processes of formulary system management.

The goal of formulary system management should be to provide sound therapeutics. To achieve this goal successfully, prescribers should be actively involved in developing the techniques used to manage the formulary system. Communication and understanding among pharmacists, prescribers, other health-care providers, and the P&T Committee members should be timely and routine. Pharmacists should ensure that a balanced presentation of drug information is provided to prescribers.

Techniques of formulary system management fall into three general categories: (1) drug use evaluation, (2) formulary maintenance, and (3) drug product selection.

1. Drug Use Evaluation

Drug use evaluation is an ongoing, structured, organizationally authorized process designed to ensure that drugs are used appropriately, safely, and effectively. A well-designed drug use evaluation program applies continuous quality improvement methods to the drug use process. The role and responsibilities of pharmacists in drug use evaluation are very well identified. Drug use evaluation is a quality-assurance activity, but it may also be considered a formulary system management technique. The P&T committee should be involved in the drug use evaluation process.

Effective drug use evaluation begins with (i) drug use criteria or (ii) treatment guidelines approved by the P&T committee on behalf of the medical staff. Drug use evaluation should measure and compare the outcomes of patients whose treatment did, or did not, comply with approved criteria or guidelines. Based on this comparative information, criteria or guidelines can be revised, compliance can be encouraged, educational programs can be initiated, or changes can be made to the formulary system. Drug use evaluation programs should include provisions for periodic review of all components of the system.

(i) Drug Use Criteria

In cases where a drug poses potential efficacy, toxicity, or utilization problems for the health-care setting, criteria may be established by the P&T committee to promote appropriate use. Drug use criteria are approved guidelines regarding how, or under what conditions, a drug is recommended for use. Preliminary drug use criteria should be developed at the time that a drug is proposed for addition to the formulary. Drug use criteria should be updated as needed over time. There are three general types of criteria: diagnosis criteria, prescriber criteria, and drug-specific criteria. Criteria of any type can be used independently or in combination.

Diagnosis criteria identify indications that constitute acceptable uses for a formulary drug within the health-care setting. Protocols, if any, for restricting the use of a formularydrug to specific diagnoses or medical conditions should be established by the P&T Committee. For instance, a particular colony-stimulating factor might be approved for use only as an adjunct to cancer chemotherapy. Use of this drug for other indications would then fall outside the approved diagnosis criteria.

Prescriber criteria identify prescribers approved to use specific formulary drugs or drug classes. Examples include limiting the use of specific injectable antibiotics to infectious disease specialists or establishing cardiologists or emergency room physicians as the only approved prescribers for thrombolytic drugs.

Drug-specific criteria identify approved doses, frequency of administration, duration of therapy, or other aspects that are specific to the use of a formulary drug. An example would be limiting the dosing of a long-acting injectable antibiotic to once every 24 hours. More frequent dosing regimens might require approval by an infectious disease specialist.

(ii) Treatment Guidelines

Treatment guidelines are similar to drug use criteria, except that treatment guidelines focus on disease-based drug therapy. Whereas drug use criteria relate to a specific drug, treatment guidelines outline a recommended therapeutic approach to specific diseases. This approach generally identifies the use of several different drugs, depending on disease severity or specific patient characteristics.

A treatment guideline, for example, may outline a recommended approach to treating community-acquired pneumonia, reflux esophagitis, or otitis media, or it may list drugs to be used in bone marrow transplantation. Treatment guidelines are typically developed and approved by P&T committees for high risk, high volume, or problem-prone diseases encountered in the health-care setting.

2. Formulary Maintenance

Formulary maintenance techniques include

- Therapeutic drug class review.
- Processes by which drug products are added to or deleted from the formulary.
- Use of non formulary drugs in unique patient situations.

To be effective in improving the drug use process, pharmacists and medical staff must work collaboratively.

The pharmacist should assume responsibility and a leadership role in the development and presentation of information required by the P&T committee for decision making. The medical staff must understand and support the processes by which these techniques are applied, as well as participate in the development and review of information.

Therapeutic Drug Class Review : It is useful for the P&T committee to review the use and therapeutic effects of several classes of drug products every year. Examples of drug classes suitable for review are nonsteroidal anti-inflammatory agents, injectable cephalosporins, antihistamines, β-blockers, and neuromuscular blockers. These reviews can be prompted by criteria set by the P&T Committee itself. For example, based on the number of adverse drug reaction reports, new information in the medical literature, or drug class expenditures, the committee can determine which classes of formulary drugs are worthy of reassessment.

The goal is to identify preferred agents based on effectiveness, toxicity, or cost differences within the same class. It is important that appropriate medical staff input, outside the committee, be solicited during these reviews. Outcomes of therapeutic class reviews can include development of new drug use criteria, new treatment guidelines, or changes to the formulary.

Formulary Addition or Deletion : Attending physicians or pharmacists may request drugs to be added to or deleted from the formulary by completing a formulary drug request form. The Pharmacy and Therapeutics Committee may initiate its own review of a drug if a number of non-formulary drug requests are received. Routine drug class reviews may also trigger formulary additions or deletions. When a drug is added to the formulary, consideration should routinely be given to deleting other items.

Drugs are added to the formulary based on objective, scientific data. Considerations include effectiveness, side effect profile, cost, medication error potential, and comparison to alternative agents, if available. Pharmacy Services staff provides an objective evidence-based medical evaluation for each drug requested for formulary addition to assist the Committee in its deliberations.The physician or pharmacist who requests the addition of a drug to the formulary may be requested to attend the Pharmacy and Therapeutics Committee meeting when it is considered.

Use of Non formulary Drugs : In general, only formulary drugs are endorsed as appropriate for *routine* use within the organized health-care setting. The underlying principle for the existence of a process for approval of non formulary drugs is that individual or unique patient needs can exist that may not be satisfied by the use of formulary drugs. There should be an approved policy and procedure for obtaining approval for use of non formulary drugs. This process should include the generation of information on the use of non formulary drugs to enable the P&T committee to review trends in non formulary drug use, which may influence formulary addition or deletion decisions. There should also be a process in place for obtaining non formulary drugs in a timely manner. In managed care settings, the decision to approve the use of non formulary drugs is separate from the decision to grant payment coverage for a drug. Coverage decisions are governed by the patient's contract with a specific health plan.

3. Drug Product Selection

Pharmacists and prescribers must understand the concept of therapeutic equivalence to ensure proper application of generic substitution and therapeutic interchange principles.

Pharmacists should assume a leadership role in drug product selection by proposing opportunities for drug product selection. This includes evaluation and assessment of bioequivalence data; storage, dispensing, and administration characteristics; cost; and other relevant product information.

Pharmacists must also ensure that products of adequate quality are procured. The application of generic substitution and therapeutic interchange principles may result in a drug product being dispensed to the patient that is different from the product originally prescribed. To ensure high quality drug therapy, therapeutic equivalence between the product dispensed and that prescribed must be ensured.

Therapeutic Equivalence : Therapeutic equivalence can serves as a guideline to assist in drug substitution between chemically identical products. Both generic substitution and therapeutic interchange, however, should be safe and effective if the therapeutic equivalence of products to be exchanged has been established. For the purpose of this document, drugs are considered therapeutically equivalent if they can be expected to produce essentially the same therapeutic outcome and toxicity. The use of therapeutically equivalent products can contribute to improvement in the drug use process by maintaining a high quality of drug therapy in the most cost effective manner.

Generic Substitution : For the purpose of this document, generic substitution is defined as the substitution of drug products that contain the same active ingredient(s) and are chemically identical in strength, concentration, dosage form, and route of administration to the drug product prescribed. These products can also be termed "generic equivalents." Logically, these products should display therapeutic equivalence. The key word in this definition is "identical." For example, the substitution of one brand of propranolol tablets for another represents the application of generic substitution if the strength of the active ingredients and the dosage form are identical. To ensure quality patient care, the two propranolol products must also be shown to achieve therapeutic equivalence as defined above. The substitution of purified pork insulin for human insulin is not generic substitution, because the products are not chemically identical. However, the interchangeability of these products may be acceptable under the principle of therapeutic interchange (discussed below), provided that therapeutic equivalence can be ensured.

Prescribers have the prerogative to override a generic substitution. In some cases, a patient preference may negate an otherwise acceptable generic substitution. The P&T Committee is responsible for determining which drugs are acceptable for generic substitution and for developing guidelines for pharmacists who carry out this formulary system management activity. Typically, pharmacists determine which products are purchased and dispensed as generic substitutes. In most healthcare settings, prescribers prospectively authorize generic substitution during their credentialing process. Notification of generic substitution is generally not provided to the prescriber at the time that a generic equivalent is dispensed.

Therapeutic Interchange : Therapeutic interchange is defined, for the purpose of this document, as the interchange of various therapeutically equivalent drug products by pharmacists under arrangements between pharmacist(s) and authorized prescriber(s) who have previously established and jointly agreed on conditions for interchanges.

Therapeutic interchange occurs pursuant to development of agreements between pharmacists & prescribers and implies that there is appropriate and timely communication between them. Therapeutic interchange agreements can vary from simple understandings to complex protocols. For example, a therapeutic interchange agreement permitting interchange between cephradine and cephalexin may be a simple arrangement; the dose and dosage form of the two drugs are equivalent, and the drugs typically can be interchanged in the treatment of any disease for which the drugs are indicated. A therapeutic interchange arrangement that permits the interchangeability of different colony-stimulating factors in treating a specific diagnosis pursuant to specific protocols might be more complex. In either case, the P&T committee acts on behalf of the medical staff to develop and approve these arrangements. The approval of a therapeutic interchange arrangement is typically a separate decision by a P&T Committee, unrelated to adding or deleting drugs from the formulary. In some settings, all drugs that may be therapeutically interchanged are acceptable to the formulary, and the pharmacy is authorized to purchase and dispense the most cost-effective products. In other settings, certain drug products are deemed interchangeable, but the P&T Committee designates a preferred product and approves it for formulary addition. Then the other equivalent drugs or products are deleted from the formulary.

To remain effective over time, therapeutic interchange decisions should be routinely reviewed and revised as appropriate. Therapeutic interchange may not be appropriate for all patients. Professional judgment must be exercised by the pharmacist and the prescriber. Consultation with the prescriber and the patient may be necessary. Prescribers have the prerogative to override a therapeutic interchange. In some cases, a patient preference may negate an otherwise acceptable therapeutic interchange. Pharmacists should strive for consistency of product use to avoid unnecessary switching of products dispensed to patients. When a change is made, the pharmacist should ensure that appropriate monitoring and follow up are undertaken to identify and prevent any unexpected or untoward patient response. The pharmacist should provide appropriate notification and educational materials to prescriber's, patients, and other health-care providers as needed regarding therapeutic interchange decisions.

9

Chapter

Drug Information Services

Due to advancement in Pharmaceutical industry, development of new dosage forms is a continuous process for the existing drug molecule or due to advancement in drug discovery process, new drug molecule is developed for the effective and safe drug therapy. New drug molecule is also developed for the treatment of complicated disease like cancer, HIV infection,etc. To know the new development, the physician has to update his knowledge. For this, the provision of accurate and timely drug information to health care professionals is an important mechanism to promote safe and effective drug therapy.

For this, there is need of Drug Information Service Center (DISC) which provides health care professionals with up-to-date, objective, clinically applicable information to ensure the safe, appropriate and cost-effective use of medications. The term 'drug information' was coined in the early sixties and the first Drug Information Center (DIC) was opened at the University of Kentucky Medical Center. This Service was conducted for the doctors in a clinical meet. Such information service center is not frequent in India

Examples of the types of medication-related information the Drug Information Service Center frequently provides to health care professionals include:

- Dosing, dosing schedule, and routes of administration
- Dosing adjustments in renal or hepatic dysfunction
- Therapeutic indications
- Drug product availability
- Drug identification (including foreign drugs)

- Adverse drug reactions and side effects
- Drug interactions (drug-drug, drug-food, drug-lab)
- Drug compatibility and stability
- Drug use during breast feeding
- Teratogenicity potential
- Pharmacokinetic information
- Therapeutic alternatives
- Investigational drug information
- General therapeutic information

Sources of Information

A drug information centre must possess a good collection of source material in order to answer the question whenever they arise. This should be continuously updated and maintained.

Information emerges originally from research and development. Such information's are publicized for the first time by way of what are 'Primary source'. Sometimes, these may take the form of informal communications and letters between persons working in the same field. Conferences including discussion and session can be a valuable source of primary information. In addition, the primary sources fall into several categories.

Primary sources of Information

Researcher's and manufacturer material :

(i) Patents contain original informations regarding the discovery of a drug or its emergence as medicine in clinical field.

(ii) Report containing scientific data is submitted to the drug authority/ commission to obtain a product licence. This information is confidential but its selected parts from data sheet content.

(iii) Scientific journals. Sone journals report research, other information on new development and express view points. The contents of these journals act as primary source of information regarding the new drug. Some journals which are useful are as follows :

(a) Drugs
(b) Drugs of future
(c) British Medical Journal
(d) Drug discovery
(e) Journal of Pharmacy and Pharmacology
(f) Journal of Pharmaceutical Sciences

Secondary Sources of Information

These are usually abstracting or indexing services which summarize the information appearing in primary sources. For example, International Pharmaceutical Abstract, Chemical Abstract, Biological Abstract, Index medicus, Medicinal and Aromatic Plant Abstract, etc. These abstracts are of three types : (i) telegraphic abstract: there is usually a string of words or description of contents, (ii) Indicative abstract: there is more information structured in sentences, (iii) the informative abstract gives more information about the subject concerned.

Formularies, Pharmacopeias and text books fall into the category of secondary information sources.

Tertiary Sources of Information

These sources does answer the problems concerned but act as a pointer to where it may be found. For example, dictionaries and encyclopedia, Merck Index can guide to medical terminology, chemical nomenclature, medical importance, etc.

Other sources

Now-a days, internet source is considered a very good source of information specially when cost of Journals are very high and becoming unaffordable. Following are the important sites from where information about drugs therapy can be obtained:-

www.google.com
www.yahoo.com
www.wikipedia.org
www.Rxdruglist.com
www.sciencedirect.com

Apart from this, most of the journals have their own site from where information can be obtained on payment basis.

Other sources also include the libraries, research associations, government bodies, information centre in industries, district analyst laboratories and poison centres which can be consulted to answer the specific problems.

Storage of informations must be readily available from the collection of source material. For this, efficient filling system is required and the document must be index and classified. There are several stages to take information; firstly 'word' retrieval in which the words that adequately describe the information can be identified. Secondly, 'reference' retrieval in which the references probably pertinent to the enquiry/question are identified. Thirdly, document retrieval itself where data and information are extracted from te documents.

Each document must be stored in some accessible place and be able to be located. It must be identifiable by some label or key representing the contents.

Drug information centre may organize a symposium or conferences or seminar in specific fields to increase the knowledge of physician through Pharmacy and Therapeutics Committe. Particular problems can also be solved by organizing a discussion panel in which drug information centre can invite the specialist of that particular field.

Drug information centre can start a poison information service to provide information regarding toxicity and its treatment round the clock.

DRUG INFORMATION BULLETIN

Drug bulletins are specialised periodicals providing comparative information and advice on the prescribing and use of medicines. Doctors and pharmacists are the primary audience for most of the drug bulletins.

The Drug Information Centre publishes a quarterly Drug Bulletin, which covers news about National Drug Policy, aspects of clinical pharmacology, pharmaceutical treatment and prevention guidelines, adverse drug reactions, etc. It is distributed free of charge to doctors, pharmacist and policymakers. Ideas for bulletin articles come from participation in the meetings of the Ministry of Health and Drug Department, requests from health professionals and the public, and from monitoring implementation of drug reform. Recent topics included features of pharmacotherapy in paediatrics, drug interactions, medical errors related to the names of drugs, and modified–release preparations of drugs.

10

Chapter

Over-the-Counter (OTC) Medications

Over-The-Counter (OTC) medications are those than can be taken without a prescription. While in the past, many OTC drugs were ineffective, but now many OTC medicines are highly potent drugs. The consumer should choose OTC drugs wisely.

The best way to assure that an OTC drug is right for you is to discuss your situation with a pharmacist. The pharmacist can evaluate your situation and decide which, if any, OTC drug is appropriate. The choice of OTC products for any condition can be confusing. For instance, hundreds of different products claim effectiveness for colds, flu, allergies, sinus conditions, while they all contain similar ingredients.

Not every condition requires medication treatment. For many mild conditions, such as colds, rest and fluids are just as effective as most OTC products. Take medications only when they are necessary. Never take any OTC medication during pregnancy without first talking with your provider.

Because OTC products may contain potent medications, they may cause side effects. They can worsen your medical conditions or cause a drug interaction. Discuss these issues with your pharmacist before purchasing an OTC product.

If you do purchase an OTC product, follow the dosage recommendations closely. If you are treating a small child, discuss the use of the product with your pediatrician. Never give an aspirin-containing product to a child with a fever.

OTC products can be helpful in treating symptoms of certain conditions. If your symptoms continue, see your health care provider.

Labeling Requirements

Increasingly consumers are practicing self-diagnosis and are self-treating with OTC drug products instead of seeing a physician. Understandable labels will help consumers choose the right medication and avoid harmful mistakes. By reading an OTC label, consumers should be able to determine if this is the appropriate drug for the condition being treated, the benefits of the drug, necessary precautions, and when to consult a pharmacist or other health professional. The Food and Drug Administration (FDA) is issuing a final rule establishing a standardized format and standardized content requirements for the labeling of over-the-counter (OTC) drug products. This final rule is intended to assist consumers in reading and understanding OTC drug product labeling so that consumers may use these products safely and effectively. This final rule will require all OTC drug products to carry the new, easy-to-read format and the revised content requirements within prescribed implementation periods.

The label/leaflet should contain following information:-

- The product name.
- Ingredients.
- Indications (what the medicine is for).
- The usual dosage and directions for use.
- Warnings (when to stop taking the medicine; when to see a doctor; possible side-effects).
- Storage condition
- Expiry date (when to throw it out).
- Batch number
- Name and address of manufacturer

Establishment of an OTC medication counter

The OTC counter is a part of medical store. The establishment of OTC counter means establishment of medical store. The medical store does the dispensing, sale and distribution of OTC medications. Some OTC drugs are placed in big medical store to attract the consumer like health related products (vitamin preparation, tonics, etc.); laxatives, contraceptive pills, cold relieving preparations, pain killers.

Various factors which should be considered before establishing a medical store are:

(i) Selection of Site

The premises may be owned or rented for lease for certain period of time. The cost of premises depends on location/city. Preferably it should be on ground floor. The site of premises should be in good business area means in big super market area, near to the hospital or near to thickly populated area. Now-a-days, it is advisable that site which is selected should have the good parking area.

(ii) Layout of Medical store

The layout/area of medical store should fulfill the requirement mentioned in the Schedule 'N' mentioned in Drug and Cosmetic Act. Apart from this, it should have big and attractive front door for easy approach, drinking water facility, and public telephone facility. There should have enough space for keeping the prescription and non prescription drugs. It is preferred to have the separate counter for OTC medication to attract the consumers.

(iii) Equipment and facilities

There should be good working equipments and appropriate facilities for the Personnel working and consumers/patients. Generally, medical store contains:

(a) adequate sale counter
(b) adequate dispensing section (it contains the sufficient number of physical/dispensing balances)
(c) sufficient waiting area
(d) drinking water facility
(e) Computerized cash counter

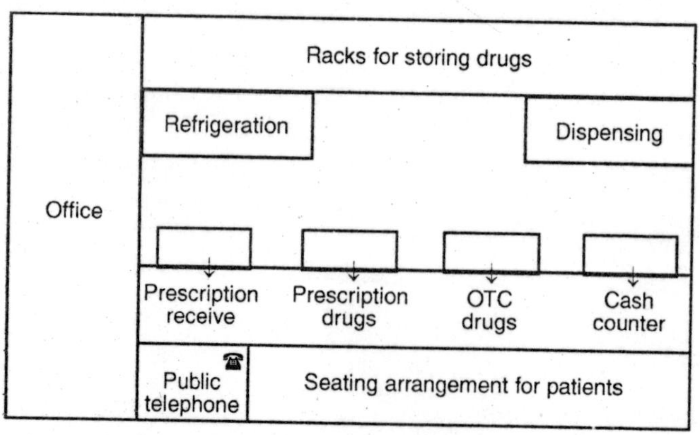

Fig. 10.1. Layout of store.

(f) Store rooms for storing the raw material and finished products
(g) Sufficient glass apparatus

(iv) Personnel

There should be adequate number of registered pharmacists, assistant pharmacist, attendants and cashier.

(v) Quality control Procedure

This is not established in India at the medical store level. The quality is just observed by seeing the label of drug, manufacture name, batch number and expiry date. The dispensing of OTC medication is done by the qualified Pharmacist and it is well documented. The documented record should contain:

(a) name of patient, age
(b) master formula and its source (I.P or B.P.)
(c) name of ingredients and the quantity of each ingredient
(d) direction of use
(e) storage condition
(f) date of dispensing

(vi) Information Bulletin

The physician is generally not involved in prescribing the OTC medication. So there should be a proper guidance about the use of OTC medication by the Pharmacist. To guide the patient, there should be sufficient information materials like the I.P., B.P., MIMS, Merck Index, etc. Presently, internet facility is a best source to take the information material about any OTC drug.

General Advice for Using OTC Drugs

(i) Use of OTC drugs during pregnancy

Over-the-counter (OTC) drugs are readily accessible, widely used and, because they can be obtained without medical advice, are often perceived as being 'safe'. Drugs in general should be avoided during pregnancy if possible. However, OTC drug usage during pregnancy is increasing because of advertising by the pharmaceutical industry and the lack of data showing the adverse effects of OTC preparations on the fetus.

An increasing number of prescription drugs are being given OTC status. Some OTC drugs are known to adversely affect the fetus but drugs for which there is a lack of clinical data may also have the potential to produce adverse fetal effects when taken during pregnancy. In addition to the active drug, excipients of OTC preparations may affect fetal development. The effects on the fetus of an interaction between two OTC products or between an OTC product and a prescribed drug also need to be considered. In addition, some medications may present more risk to the fetus according to the stage of gestation (e.g. many medications are potentially harmful in the first trimester but pose less risk later in pregnancy). Pregnant women should be advised to consult a pharmacist or doctor before using any OTC medication.

Similarly, breast-feeding mother should consult the pharmacist before taking OTC drug as drugs may enter the breast milk and inadvertently pass to the nursing baby as well.

(ii) Use of OTC drugs by Children

Teens are taking Over-The-Counter pain relievers and cough & cold medicines just to get high. And they are getting them easily from their own homes, or the homes of other relatives and friends. In fact, nearly half (47%) of teens say they get these drugs for free from a relative or friend. Ten percent say they buy pain relievers from a friend or relative, and another 10 percent say they took drugs without asking. It is sort of abuse which is difficult to monitor. Only the parents can do it by observing them.

(iii) Chronic use of OTC drugs

Just because a medicine is available over the counter does not mean it is completely safe, and you should always check with your doctor before taking it. Moreover, sometimes OTC drugs can actually be harmful. For example, taking painkillers over many years can cause kidney failure and swallowing tablets to self-treat a fever may mask certain illnesses such as tuberculosis or malaria. Similarly, consumption of OTC medicines over a long period can create new problems: for example, totals dependence on laxatives or sleeping pills. Self-medication can be sensible and beneficial, but only if done intelligently. Don't just depend on a friend's advice or on your chemist's suggestions: always discuss OTC drugs with your doctor/Pharmacist.

(iv) *Use of OTC drugs with Prescription drugs*

Certain OTC drugs may affect the way your body reacts to the prescription drugs you are taking. For instance, people taking tetracycline should avoid taking antacids at the same time because the latter interfere with the body's absorption of the former, thereby decreasing its effectiveness. Consequently, you must know precisely what OTC drugs you are taking, and let your doctor/Pharmacist know as well.

Nowadays, many homeopathic and ayurvedic medicines are also available over the counter as well. Don't automatically assume that because these medicines are 'natural' they are completely safe – remember that every medicine can have side-effects. You should apply the same common-sense principles to OTC medicines that you do to all other medicines.

(v) Miscellaneous

Unfortunately, the leaflet/label of OTC drugs will not tell you everything you need to know about using OTC drugs, in part because manufactures don't want to keep their customers away. You can get complete information only by asking your doctor. Read the package insert or label before you leave the store, so that you can ask the pharmacist to clarify anything that you don't understand.

Here are some rules to follow when taking OTC drugs :

(a) Take the least amount of drug possible to get the desired effect.

(b) Use multi symptom medications (which contain a mixture of many drugs) only if you have all the symptoms that they treat. The more the active ingredients in the medicine, the higher the risk of adverse reactions and interactions.

(c) Take most OTC drugs either one hour before or two hours after eating, to prevent food from reducing their absorption and effectiveness.

(d) Never mix alcohol and medications.

(e) If a problem doesn't get better, worsens, or clears up and then returns, see a doctor. Some medications can make symptoms worse if take far too long.

(f) Check label dates before buying or using medications.

11
Chapter

Medical Stores

Medical Stores in Hospitals is responsible is responsible ensuring continuous distribution of Pharmaceutical products in a financially viable and sustainable manner. In addition, Medical stores distributes drugs and various other items which currently include Essential Drug Kits and Family Planning Products.

The Objectives of Medical Stores

The following are the principal objectives of the corporation :

- Efficient and economic procurement of medicines and certain other medical supplies of good quality primarily to the public health services.
- Secure safe and efficient storage, administration, distribution and supply of goods in question in accordance to the National Drug Policy and Authority.
- Establishment and maintenance of systems to ensure the quality of goods supplied.
- Estimation of current and future needs as a basis for procurement, planning and budgeting by the corporation itself and the Ministries concerned.

In fulfilling the above objectives, Medical Stores has the following advantages as an autonomous centralized drug supplier:

- ***Cost effectiveness*** : Central procurement of essential drugs is the most cost-effective method for the public sector because the discounts attained through bulk procurement are translated into affordable prices to the end user.

Quality assurance : Under central procurement there are fewer chances of importing sub standard drugs and in rare cases where they do, mechanisms have been put in place to ensure immediate recall.

- *Financing* : After the initial one-time capital investment the system became self-sustaining.

Layout of Medical Store

The layout of medical stores should have :

(i) the Central Medical Stores (CMS) administrative building
(ii) the Pharmacy Board Offices,
(iii) the Quality Control Laboratory
(iv) receipt section
(v) storage section (separate for drugs and health accessories)
(vi) issue section
(vii) record rooms

(i) The CMS administrative building comprising

- 1 meeting room
- 1 directorial office with rest room
- 1 Executive Secretary office
- 1 waiting room
- 5 Deputy Directors offices
- 10 agent offices
- 1 computerising room
- 1 cashier room
- 1 telephone room
- 1 reception room
- 1 samples room

(ii) The storage section

The storage section assessed during the inception phase must be high enough to allow the putting in of pallet loaders and the storage on three levels, and wide enough to allow the storage on four rows of pallets and further the use inside of a fork lift, in order to increase threefold the storage capacity.

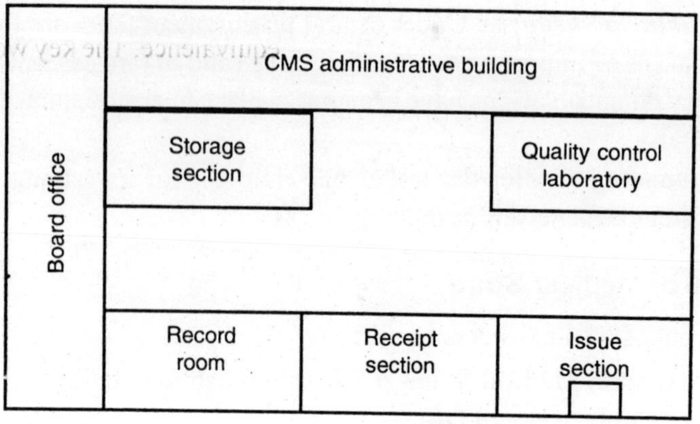

Fig. 11.1a. Layout for medical store.

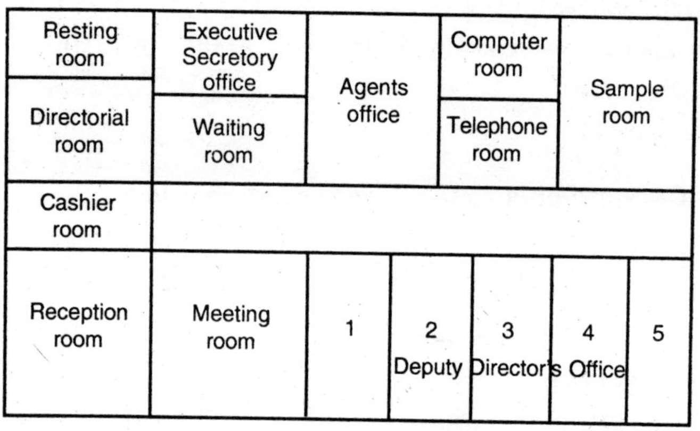

Fig. 11.1b. Layout for CMS administrative building.

The warehouse must have :

- a receiving bay for the containers
- a quarantine store space able to store drugs or medical supplies of three containers of 40 feet
- a storage space for the storage of drugs of 15 containers of 40 feet
- a cold store of 6 mL × 4 mW × 4 mH capacity
- a dispatching store for drugs delivery
- a dispatching bay for the tucks of ten tones

The Expert will propose a drawing of that storage section taking into account international rules of safety and ventilation for warehouses.

(iii) The Pharmacy Board and the Quality Control Laboratory

It consist of :

- ***For the Pharmacy Board***
  - 1 Executive office with rest room
  - 1 Executive Secretary office
  - 1 waiting room
  - 4 offices
  - 1 reception
  - 1 conference hall
  - 1 library
  - 4 rest rooms
- ***For the Quality Control Laboratory***
  - 1 storage room
  - 1 laboratory with four units
  - 3 rest rooms

PROCUREMENT OF DRUGS AND SUPPLIES

The method of procuring drugs depends on size of hospitals as well as type of hospitals. Generally big sized hospitals would like to take drugs and supplies directly from the manufacturer through tendering process. Government hospitals take most of the medicines from the central medical store depot. The small sized hospitals take the medicines and supplies from distributer or retailer. Whatever the hospital, generally there are four strategic objectives of pharmaceutical procurement.

Four Strategic Objectives of Pharmaceutical Procurement

(a) Procure the most cost-effective drugs in the right quantities

The first strategic objective is that all organizations responsible for procurement, whether they are public, private non-profit or private for-profit, should develop an essential drugs list to make sure that only the most cost-effective drugs are purchased. Procedures must also be in place that accurately estimates procurement quantities in order to ensure continuous access to the products selected without accumulating excess stock.

(b) Select reliable suppliers of high-quality products

The second objective is that reliable suppliers of high-quality products must be pre-selected, and that active quality assurance programmes involving both surveillance and testing must be implemented.

(c) Ensure timely delivery

The third strategic objective is that the procurement and distribution systems must ensure timely delivery of appropriate quantities to central or provincial stores and adequate distribution to health facilities where the products are needed.

(d) Achieve the lowest possible total cost

The fourth objective is that the procurement and distribution systems must achieve the lowest possible total cost, considering four main components :

- the actual purchase price of drugs;
- hidden costs due to poor product quality, poor supplier performance or short shelf-life;
- inventory holding costs at various levels of the supply system; and
- operating costs and capital loss by management and administration of the procurement and distribution system.

Procurement from Medical Store Depot

Govt. Medical Store Depot (GMSD) is functioning under Medical Stores Organization which is a subordinate office of Ministry of Health & F.W., Govt. of India. Many Medical store depot exist in different cities in India like Delhi, Chennai, Kolkatta, Karnal, Hyderabad, Gauhati, etc. The main functions and duties of the GMSDs are as under:

(i) To procure and supply medicines, surgical equipments and other medical stores required by the hospitals and dispensaries etc. run by Central Govt., para-military forces and CGHS etc.

(ii) Receipt, storage and distribution of supplies of drugs and allied stores including vaccines received from WHO, UNICEF, USAID and under the various international bodies under various agreements entered into by the Govt. of India.

(iii) Storage and issue of stores required under various National Health & F.W. programmes including Anti-TB, Anti-Leprosy, NMEP,

RCH etc. throughout the country (10 States i.e. Haryana, Punjab, Himachal Pradesh, Jammu & Kashmir,Rajasthan, UT Chandigarh, Delhi, Uttranchal, Uttar Pradesh and some part of Bihar and Madhya Pradesh so far as GMSD, Karnal is concerned).

(iv) Meeting the emergency requirements of life saving drugs and other allied items in the country, arising out of natural calamities such as floods, cyclones, droughts, riots etc. and other national calamities.

The Government hospitals/CGHS dispensories usually procure most of the medicine from medical store depot. They quantify their needs and send to the medical store depot in the indent form in the early financial year. The medical store depot do the procuring job and time to time send the medicine to these hospital/dispensaries.

Procurement from Manufacturer/Distributors

Procurement Procedure : This procedure is applicable when the drugs and supplies has to procured from the manufacturer or distributer. It is observed in India, distributer is involved when the drug and supplies have to be imported. In most of the situation, manufacturer do not supply, they sell their items through the distributer appointed for India, It may be due to involvement of lot of Government formalities.

The procurement procedure broadly consists of the following steps :

1. Assessment of requirement
2. Deciding procurement strategy including technical specifications
3. Mode of procurement
4. Preparation of tender document
5. Advertisement of the tender
6. Issue of tender documents
7. Opening of the tender
8. Evaluation of the tender
9. Clearance of World Bank/DFID, whenever required
10. Award of contract
11. Notification of delivery to consignee
12. Inspection and testing
13. Receipt of consignment
14. Acceptance and storage of the consignment.
15. Resolution of disputes, if any

1. Assessment of the Requirement

Bulk requirement of the stores at state level/district level should be assessed prior to the beginning of the financial year to get the competitive prices and action for procurement should be initiated in accordance with the purchase procedures. While forecasting the requirement, the following factors should be considered:

- Average time period required in complete procurement cycle. In some cases, it can take 8 to 12 months to complete the procurement cycle.
- The trends in usage at the time of requirement.
- Current stock of the store, where is the stock located, when is the product due to reach the expiry date and what is the projected time scale for distribution.
- Storage capacity for receiving the bulk consignment. In case the storage capacity is limited, it would be required that the procurement/supply of commodities be phased over time rather than arriving as one consignment.
- List of consignees and their storage capacity.
- The problem, if any, encountered with the procurement and distribution over the last few years.

Consolidating several programme procurement requirements can offer potential savings through price discounts and reduces the purchaser's administrative cost associated with having to process multiple orders.

2. Deciding on Procurement Strategy

It is important to agree on the procurement strategy before initiating the tendering. For example purchase of drugs having limited life shall require different procurement strategy than purchase of say hospital beds. Issues like pre-qualification of suppliers to reduce the procurement cycle time in case of life saving drugs and having multiple supply lines for essential items should also be considered. Similarly for civil works, options like work contract on lump-sum basis or based on bill of quantities can be explored. The procurement strategy should cover :

- key objectives of the procurement for the project;
- chosen procurement option;
- chosen procurement route (open, restricted);

- key milestones (check that enough time will be allowed for various procurement steps);
- key documents e.g. requirements specification.

3. Mode of Procurement

The methods of procurement normally followed are:

A. Global tender/International Competitive Bidding (ICB)
B. Open advertised tender/National Competitive Bidding (NCB)
C. Limited Tender (National/International)
D. Shopping (National/International)
E. Single tender/Direct Contracting

(A) **Global tender/International Competitive Bidding (ICB):** This method is generally adopted where the supplies need import and foreign firms are expected to participate irrespective of the value.

(B) **Open advertised tender/National Competitive Bidding (NCB):**

(i) Open tender is the competitive bidding procedure normally used for public procurement in the country and may be the most efficient and economic way of procuring goods or works, by their nature or scope. The procedures shall provide for adequate competition in order to ensure reasonable prices. The method to be used in the evaluation of tenders and the award of contracts shall be made known to all bidders and not be applied arbitrarily.

(ii) Open tender is the normally adopted method of procurement.

(iii) *Notification/advertising* : Timely notification of bidding opportunities is essential in competitive bidding :

(a) Invitation to bid shall be published in daily newspapers with wide circulation all over India, at least in one national english and one regional language daily. If the advertisement is for more than one item, it should also be indicated whether the evaluation would be item-wise or as a package. The bidders shall be allowed the option to submit the bids for any one or more items. The advertisement should also be placed at the website of the department.

(b) If it is a condition in the invitation for tender that Earnest Money (it should be a specific amount rather than a %) is to be deposited by the supplier/contractor, the bid of a supplier/contractor not complying with this requirement, shall be rejected.

(c) In a package, the ernest money is indicated taking into account all the items. This cannot be changed later on.

(d) The last date for receipt of tender shall be the day following the date for close of the sale of tender documents.

(e) Tendering period shall not be less than 30 days from the date of start of sale of tender documents.

(f) Tenders can be sold from different places but the tenders shall be received at one place to avoid problems arising out of late/delayed tenders. Tenders should normally be opened immediately after the deadline for receipt time.

(iv) *Tender documents* : Sale of tender document should begin only after the publication of notification for tender in newspaper. The tender documents shall furnish all information necessary for a prospective bidder to prepare a tender for the goods and works to be provided. Tender documents should be made available to all who seek them after paying the requisite fees, if any, regardless of registration status and they should be allowed to bid.

(v) *Clarity of tender documents* : Tender documents shall furnish clearly and precisely for the work to be carried out, the location of the work, the goods to be supplied, the place of delivery or installation, the schedule for delivery or completion, specification/technical specification, minimum performance requirements, the warranty and maintenance requirements, if any, and the method of evaluation. The basis for tender evaluation and selection of the lowest technically suitable and evaluated tender shall be clearly outlined in the instructions to tenders and/or the specifications. Tender documents should state clearly whether the bid prices will be fixed or price adjustments will be made to reflect any changes in major cost components of the contract.

(vi) *Standards and technical specifications* : The implementing agency shall specify the generally accepted standards of technical specifications. Unbiased technical specification shall be prepared with no mention of brand names and catalogue numbers. In case the item to be procured is not covered under I.P., specifications are to be framed, specifications may be prepared by a committee of experts associating the trade, if required. The functional performance, design, quality, packaging and additional requirements should be clearly spelt out in the specifications. The specifications should be generic and should not appear to favour a particular brand or supplier. Technical specifications, bill of quantities and civil drawings should be prepared before tendering. Specifications for the articles to be procured should be drawn up in every case with clarity. No deviations from the specifications after opening of tender should be allowed.

(vii) *Validity of tender* : Bidders shall be required to submit tender valid for the period specified in the tender documents. Normally, the bid validity period shall not exceed 90 days.

(viii) *Ernest money* : Ernest money of normally 2% of the estimated cost of the item or works shall be the appropriate amount, which should be indicated, in a specific amount. The earnest money shall be in the form of a demand draft/banker's cheque/ bank guarantee from a scheduled bank, which should be valid up to 45 days beyond the validity period of the tender. The earnest money of unsuccessful bidders shall be refunded soon after the final acceptance of tenders. The earnest money shall be forfeited in the event of withdrawal of the tender within the original validity once submitted or in case a successful bidder fails to execute necessary agreement within the period specified.

(ix) *Pre bid conference* : A pre-bid conference (date/venue to be indicated in the bid document) may be arranged wherein potential bidders may meet with the representatives of the implementing authority to seek clarifications on the tender documents. Copy of minutes of the pre-bid conference should be furnished to the bidders who had already purchased the bid documents and also along with the bid document sold to the parties purchasing the document subsequent to the pre-bid conference.

(x) *Terms and methods of payment* : Payment terms shall be in accordance with the practices applicable to the specific goods and works. Tender documents should specify the payment method and terms offered.

(xi) *Conditions of contract* : The contract documents shall clearly define the scope of work to be performed, the goods to be supplied, the rights and obligations of the implementing agency and of the supplier or contractor, and the functions and authority of the engineer, architect, or construction manager, (if one is employed by the implementing agency) in the supervision and administration of the contract. Special conditions related to specific item should also be clearly specified in the tender document.

(xii) *Performance security deposit* :

(a) Tender documents for works and goods shall require security in an amount sufficient to protect the implementing agency in case of breach of contract by the contractor. This shall be in the form of a bank guarantee or any other instrument and amount should be specified in the tender document. The amount of performance guarantee shall normally be 5% of contract price (valid till 28 days from the date of expiry of defect liability period or the guarantee/warranty period as the case may be).

(b) The performance security deposit shall be refunded within one month of the completion of supply of goods/works. It will, however, be refunded after the expiry of guarantee/warranty period (as mentioned above) where there is condition of guarantee/warrantee.

(c) The performance security deposit shall be forfeited in case any terms and conditions of the contract are infringed or the bidder fails to make complete supply satisfactorily or complete the work within the delivery/completion period agreed in the contract.

(xiii) *Retention money* : In contracts for works, normally 5-10% of contract price shall be recovered for retention money. 50% of such retention money shall be retained till completion of the whole of the works and 50% shall be retained till the end of defects liability period.

(xiv) *Liquidated damages* : Provisions for liquidated damages shall be included in the conditions of contract when delays in the delivery of goods, completion of works would result in extra cost, or loss of revenue or loss of other benefits or inconvenience to the implementing agency.

(xv) *Tender opening* :

- The time for the tender opening should be immediately after the deadline for receipt time as discussed above.
- Tenders shall be opened in public. The bidders or their representatives shall be allowed to be present at the time of opening of bids.
- All tenders received should be opened. No bid should be rejected at bid opening except for late tenders. Late tenders shall be returned to the bidders unopened.
- The name of the bidder and total amount of each bid along with important conditions like excise duty, sales tax, delivery terms, delivery period, special conditions, if any, shall be read out at the time of bid opening.
- Spot comparative statement (minutes of bid opening) must be prepared by the bid opening official and should be signed.

(xvi) *Confidentiality* : After the public opening of tenders, information relating to the examination, clarification, and evaluation of tenders and recommendations concerning awards shall not be disclosed to bidders or other persons not officially concerned with this process until the successful bidder is notified of the award of the contract.

(xvii) *Examination of tenders* :

(a) The implementing agency shall ascertain whether the tenders :

- Meet the eligibility requirements specified;
- Have been properly signed;
- Are accompanied by the required earnest money and valid for the period specified in the tender document;
- Are substantially responsive to the tender documents; and
- Have the technical and financial capability to successfully execute the contract. For ensuring financial capacity a minimum turnover requirement should be indicated in bid document.

(b) If a bid is not substantially responsive, that is, it contains material deviations from or reservations to the terms, conditions, and specifications in the tender documents, it shall not be considered further. The bidder shall not be permitted to correct or withdraw material deviations or reservations once tenders have been opened.

(xviii) *Tender evaluation and comparison* :

(a) The purpose of tender evaluation is to determine the cost to the implementing agency of each tender in a manner that permits a comparison based on its evaluation cost. The tender with the lowest evaluated cost and substantially responsive, but not necessarily the lowest submitted price, should be selected for award.

(b) The bid price read out at the bid opening shall be adjusted to correct any arithmetical errors for the purpose of evaluation.

(c) Evaluation of tenders should be made strictly in terms of the provisions in the tender documents to ensure compliance with the commercial and technical aspects.

(d) The conditional discounts offered by the bidder shall not be taken into account for evaluation.

(e) The past performance of the suppliers/contractors should also be taken into account while evaluating the tenders. (this should also be indicated in bid document)

(f) The implementing agency shall prepare a detailed report on the evaluation and comparison of tenders setting forth the specific reasons on which the recommendation is based for the award of the contract.

(xix) *Negotiation* : There should not be any negotiation. Negotiations if at all shall be an exception and only in the case of proprietary items. Negotiations shall be held only with the lowest evaluated responsive bidder (L-I). In case of L-1 backing out, there should be re-tendering as per extent instructions.

(xx) *Extension of validity of tenders* : As far as possible contract should be finalized with in the original validity of the offers mentioned in the tender. An extension of bid validity, if justified by exceptional circumstances with the approval of next higher authority, shall be requested in writing from all bidders (of valid tenders only) before the expiry date. Bidders shall have the right to refuse to grant such an extension without forfeiting their ernst money, but those who are willing to extend the validity of their bid shall also be required to provide a suitable extension of ernst money.

(xxi) *Post-qualification of bidders* : If bidders have not been pre-qualified, the implementing agency shall determine whether the bidder whose bid has been determined to offer the lowest evaluated cost has the technical capability and financial resources to effectively carry out the contract as offered in the bid. The criteria to be met shall be set out in the tender documents, and if the bidder does not meet them, the bid shall be rejected. In such an event, the implementing agency shall make a similar determination for the next-lowest evaluated bidder and so on.

(xxii) *Repeat orders (goods/equipment)* : Quantities in contracts awarded may be increased/decreased as per the prevailing State procedure up to 15% of the quantity originally ordered by repeat orders after recording reasons provided that such orders shall be given before the date of the expiry of last supply and also subject to the condition that prices have since not reduced and purchases were required on urgency basis.

(xxiii) *Rejection of all tenders* :

(a) The implementing agency may reject all tenders. Rejection of all tenders is justified when none of the tenders are substantially responsive or when negotiations with the L1 bidder have failed. However, lack of competition shall not be determined solely on the basis of the number of bidders. If all tenders are rejected, the implementing agency shall review the causes justifying the rejection and consider making revisions to the conditions of contract, design and specifications, scope of the contract, or a combination of these, before inviting new tenders.

(b) If the rejection of all tenders is due to lack of competition, wider advertising shall be considered. If the rejection is due to most or all of the tenders being non responsive, new tenders may be invited.

(c) Rejection of all tenders and re-inviting new tenders, irrespective of value shall be referred to the competent authority for approval after examining whether technical specifications need any change.

(C) **Limited tender (national/international) :** Limited tendering is nothing but inviting bids from qualified suppliers as per the approved list and other known suppliers broad enough to ensure receipt of competitive bids. This method shall be used only in exceptional circumstances.This procedure could be adopted where

- There are only a limited number of suppliers of the particular goods or services
- Demand is urgent in nature

(D) **Shopping :**

(a) Shopping is a procurement method based on comparing price quotations obtained from several suppliers, usually at least three to ensure competitive prices.

(b) Goods including drugs and equipment, and civil works estimated to cost the financial ceiling prevailing in states or less per contract

(c) It is an appropriate method for procuring readily available shelf goods of standard specifications commodities of small value or simple civil works of small value.

(d) Approval of competent authority may be obtained for items to be purchased or civil works to be constructed/renovated/ repaired along with specifications, estimated costs and agencies from whom quotations should be invited.

(e) The requests for quotations shall be made indicating the description, specification, and quantity of the goods, terms of delivery or specifications of works, as well as desired delivery or completion of time and place. If the quotations are called for more than one item/works, it should also be indicated whether the evaluation would be for each item-wise or for civil works or as a package.

(f) Quotations could also be obtained by telex or facsimile. The terms of the accepted offer shall be incorporated in a purchase order or brief contract.

(g) Rate contracts entered into by Directorate General of Supplies and Disposal (DGS&D) will be acceptable for procurement under shopping.

(E) **Single tender /Direct contracting :**

(a) The single tender system may be adopted in case of articles including drugs and equipment, which are specifically certified as of proprietary in nature, or where only a particular firm is the manufacturer of the articles demanded or in case of extreme emergency.

(b) The single tender system without competition shall be an appropriate method under the following circumstances:
   (i) extension of existing contracts for works or goods awarded with the prescribed procedures, justifiable on economic grounds;
   (ii) standardization of equipment or spare parts to be compatible with existing equipment may justify additional purchases from the original supplier;
   (iii) the required item is proprietary and obtainable only from one source;
   (iv) need for early delivery to avoid costly delays;
   (v) works are small and scattered or in remote locations where mobilization costs for contractors would be unreasonably high; and
   (vi) in exceptional cases, such as in response to natural disasters.

4. Award of Contract

Implementing agency shall award the contract, within the period of the validity of tenders, to the bidder who meets the tender conditions in all aspects, has the necessary technical capability and financial resources and whose bid is substantially responsive to the tender documents and has the lowest evaluated cost. The purchaser can, if so desired depute a team of 3-4 officers to the premises of manufacturer to whom the contract is proposed to be awarded, to satisfy itself that the manufacturer has capability to produce the required quantity and also the necessary quality testing and assurance facilities to meet the required standards. Based on the report of this committee, the purchaser may decide to award the contract to the successful bidder offering the lowest or reasonable price after approval of the appropriate authority. Single bids should also be considered for award, if it is determined that publicity was adequate, bid specification/conditions were not restrictive or unclear and bid prices are considered reasonable.

5. Inspection, Sampling and Testing Procedure

The inspection authority and procedure for sampling and testing should be clearly specified in the tender document. The purchaser must select a set of accredited testing laboratories for testing the samples and choose an inspection agent qualified to conduct random sampling in accordance with ISO requirements. The purchaser should request a written confirmation from the supplier that the results of the testing laboratory chosen for qualification and compliance testing will be accepted by the supplier. The name of the testing lab should be incorporated in the tender document. The authority to collect random samples should be specified. The purchaser may require verification of the WHO GMP certification of the supplier, for all procurement of pharmaceuticals. If the stores do not meet the performance requirement, they should not be accepted. If there are any disputes or doubts about the quality of the products, a procedure of resolution of dispute may be followed as per the terms of the contract. A suitable inspection agency may be hired to ensure adherence to the laid down quality standards.

6. Notification of Delivery to Consignee

Notification of delivery or dispatch in regard to each and every installment shall be made by the supplier to the purchase officer. The supplier shall further supply to the consignee a packing account quoting number of supply order and the date of dispatch of the stores. All packages, containers, bundles and loose materials part of each and every installment shall be fully described in the packing account and full details of the contents of the packages and quantity of materials shall be given to enable the consignee to check the stores on arrival at destination. The railway receipt, consignment note or the bill of the lading, if any, should be drawn in the name of the consignee and should be sent to him by registered post acknowledgement due immediately on dispatch of stores, quoting the No.(s) and date(s) of the corresponding inspection note(s) in relation to the stores covered by the said railway receipt, the consignment note or the bill of lading, as the case may be. The contractor shall bear and reimburse to the purchaser, demurrage charges, if any paid by the reasons of delay on the part of the supplier in forwarding the railway receipt, consignment note or bill of lading.

7. Receipt of Consignment

In case of imported items, the purchaser should be aware of the custom clearance requirement prior to issuing the contract. A clear procedure (i.e. who will clear the goods and pay the duties, loading and unloading of the consignment, transport of the consignment to the premises of the consignee etc.) for custom clearance should be specified in the contract.

At the time of the delivery of the stores, the consignee should accept the items on "said to contain" basis and should issue the provisional receipt certificate in the standard format. After opening the packages and detailed examination of the items the consignee will issue the final acceptance certificate if he is satisfied with the quality of the goods. Notwithstanding the pre-qualification or the inspection of the goods/services by the inspection agency, consignee has the right to further inspect and test the goods but within a reasonable time (say up to 60 days) and if the goods fails to meet the specifications given in the contract, he should reject the goods and ask the supplier to replace the goods or rectify the defects.

8. Storage

Experience has demonstrated that properly packed, good quality goods (except some drugs and vaccines or specific items) do not deteriorate when stored at average temperatures found in tropical climates. Air-conditioning is generally not necessary if the goods are properly packaged and stored in a clean, dry and well-ventilated environment.

If quality assurance measures have been strictly followed during the manufacturing process the conditions of warehousing and storage play a major role in ensuring that quality goods received reach final users in good condition. They should be left in their original packaging while in storage. The batch number and marking on the cartons should be recorded to ensure that every batch is traceable and distributed on a first in first expiry basis. The drugs, which require special storage including maintaining proper temperature should be stored in appropriate condition.

9. Resolution of Disputes

The dispute resolution methodology should be very clearly indicated in the contract document. As far as possible, disputes may be resolved with mutual agreement between purchaser and buyer through alternate dispute resolution methods to avoid going through arbitration and litigation stage.

There are a number of possible causes of disputes during the execution of contract. These may involve :

- interpretation of the terms and conditions of the contract
- delay in delivery/completion of the works
- delay in release of payment
- independent laboratory test results
- condition of the items on arrival at consignee and after delivery
- rate of the items, variation in quantity in civil works contract etc.
- Design/specification issues.

10. Laws Governing the Contract

(i) The contract shall be governed by the laws of India in force.

(ii) The courts of the place from where the acceptance of tender has been issued shall alone have jurisdiction to decide any dispute arising out of or in respect of the contract.

(iii) Irrespective of the place of delivery, the place of performance or place of payment under the contract or the place of issue of advance intimation of acceptance of tender, the contract shall be deemed to have been made at the place from where the acceptance of the tenders have been issued.

11. Arbitration

In the event of any question, dispute or difference arising under the contract conditions or any special conditions of contract, or in connection with the contract (except as to any matters the decision of which is specially provided for by these or the special conditions) the same shall be referred to the sole arbitrary officer, from the department other than the department who has decided the contract having sufficient knowledge of law, appointed to be the arbitrator by the purchaser. The award of the arbitrator shall be final and binding on the parties to this contract.

12. Extension of Contract (Works)

Normally a contract once awarded should not be extended. Under exceptional circumstances, extension of existing contracts up to 50% of the original contract value may be considered, if it is justifiable on economic grounds.

Procurement of Drugs from Local Market

The drugs and supplies are procured from the local market in emergency cases or when the same drug/supplies are not available in the hospital or dispensaries. The hospital approves some medical store on the basis of cost comparison. Then, particular item which are not available can be procured from the market. In some cases, the indent forms are prepared in the triplicate; one copy is given to the patient who can procure directly from that particular medical store. In every cases, the bill is reimbursed to that medical store from the hospital.

Emergency Purchases

As a general rule, the requesting department will be responsible for determining product requests which are to be classified as an emergency. Examples of emergency purchases are:

(i) the replacement of an x-ray tube which burns out,

(ii) the request for a part to repair a piece of equipment which is giving support to a patient,

(iii) the request for a product, unavailable from current inventories, which is needed to treat a trauma patient,

(iv) the acquisition of a pharmaceutical product deemed necessary to the well-being of a patient in a traumatic situation.

Since the purchasing department/committee is responsible to provide procurement support for emergency requests and since Purchasing personnel will be required to judge the authenticity of an emergency request; the following guidelines are established :

A. Departments may arrange for the emergency delivery of products outside of regular working hours, provided they notify the Purchasing Department on the next regular working day. Purchasing will then arrange for a purchase order to be issued.

B. Emergency purchases which arise during regular working hours are to be arranged through the Purchasing Department. Once contacted, Purchasing will issue a purchase order to the vendor who can respond most expeditiously. The responsible buyer will do his/her best to ensure the costs involved in making sure the purchases are reasonable with respect to existing market and/or contract conditions.

C. If the purchase department has reason to believe that the request can be accommodated by use of normal procurement practices, they are required to inform the requesting individual and provide guidance and direction as to the process which is to be used. Any disputes or disagreements which arise with the requesting individual are to be reported to the purchasing coordinator or the director of Hospital Purchasing for assistance or confirmation that the course of action taken is appropriate.

D. Every Hospital organization has some limit or emergency purchase. The limit for emergency purchase depends depend on size of Hospital or type of Hospital. For example, the limit for emergency purchase may be Rs. 5000/ for small hospital but it is more in cardiac caring Hospital. All requests exceeding limits processed as emergency purchases must be followed with a requisition from the requesting department and appropriate written documentation defining the emergency nature of the request. The documentation is to be signed by the requesting department director for purchases exceeding that limit. Documentation must include the signature of an associate administrator for purchases which exceed the limit. If documentation does not accompany the requisition or the documentation is not signed by the department director, the responsible buyer will complete and send an "Emergency Order Memorandum" to the department director for his/her signature of authorization. The responsible buyer will then track the memorandum and complete the "Emergency Order Tracking Log" appropriately. If no response has been received from the department director within a one week period, the responsible buyer will send another "Emergency Order Memorandum." This procedure is to be followed until three memorandums have been sent. The buyer is to record the actions and outcomes on the "Emergency Order Tracking Log." Photocopies of log sheets representing monthly activity are to be submitted to the purchasing coordinator for review at the end of each month.

E. Emergency purchase requests which exceed the limit are to be reviewed and authorized by the purchasing coordinator or the director of Hospital Purchasing prior to processing. In the absence of both the purchasing coordinator and the director of Hospital Purchasing, the responsible buyer is to proceed using his/her best judgment, notifying the purchasing coordinator or director of Hospital Purchasing at the next available opportunity.

12

Chapter

Maintenance of Records

The hospital is a complex organization where multiple types of activities occur. It has to keep the records of every activity. There are various type of records some of which are mentioned here.

1. Patient, Employee and Hospital Related Records

Patient record

Hospital or other rehabilitation centers shall keep adequate records, including admission and discharge notes, histories (allergic condition, family history, etc.), results of examinations, nurses' notes, social service records, records of tests performed, and other records as indicated. All records shall be written, dated and signed in an indelible manner and made a part of the patient's permanent record.

All patient medical records shall be filed in a manner which will facilitate easy retrieval of any individual's record. If records are filed according to a number system, alphabetical cross-indexing shall be available.

Records of patients are the physical property of the hospital and responsibility for control of them shall rest with the chief executive officer and governing authority.

Records and information regarding patients shall be confidential. Access to these records shall be determined by the governing authority of the facility. Inspectors for licensure or other persons authorized by State or Federal Laws shall be permitted to review medical records as necessary for compliance.

Medical records shall be preserved, either in the original or by microfilm for a period of not less than five years following the most recent discharge, or three years after the patient becomes of age.

Case Records

A Committee of professional staff members shall review quarterly a sample of active and closed records to determine compliance and effectiveness of established programs and procedures.

Case records shall contain sufficient information to identify the patient clearly, to justify the diagnosis(es) and treatment, and to document the results accurately. Required information shall, as a minimum, include:

(i) Documented evidence of the assessment of the needs of the patient, of an appropriate plan of care, and of the care and services provided.
(ii) Identification data, consent forms, and name and address of sponsor/guardian.
(iii) Medical history.
(iv) Report of physical examination, if appropriate.
(v) Observations and progress notes from each service involved.
(vi) Evaluation reports, reports of treatment and clinical findings.
(vii) Discharge summary.

Personnel Records

The facility shall maintain a personnel record for each employee. As a minimum the record shall include :

(i) Application for employment that contains information regarding education, experience, and if applicable, registration and/or licensure information of the applicant.
(ii) Record of physical examination or certificate of freedom from communicable disease.

Accounting System

The facility shall establish an accounting system which properly accounts for all revenue and expenses.

Fees

Fees for services shall be established and be made known to patients prior to, or at time of, entry into any program offered.

Hospital activities records

Each facility shall establish policies and appropriate safeguards to ensure confidentiality, protection from unauthorized removal, protection from fire and water hazards, and limit access to those authorized by the Chief Executive Officer. Records shall be maintained for a minimum of five years. Records shall include :

1. Minutes of governing body meetings.
2. Minutes of administrative and professional staff meetings.
3. Safety and health related inspection reports.
4. Financial records.
5. Accident and incident reports which shall be recorded on a form designed for this purpose and which have documentation contained thereon which indicates a thorough investigation of the accident/incident has been conducted. These reports shall apply to patients and staff members.
6. Statistical records and correspondence files.
7. Cleaning and disinfecting of therapy equipment.
8. Machine calibration.

Disposition of Records

When a hospital ceases to operate, either voluntarily or by revocation of its license, the governing body (licensee) at or prior to such action shall develop a proposed plan for the disposition of its medical records. Such plans shall be submitted to the State Committee of Public Health for approval and shall contain provisions for the proper storage, safeguarding and confidentiality, transfer and/or disposal of patient's medical records and x-ray files. Any hospital that fails to develop a plan of disposition, acceptable by the State Committee of Public Health, of its records shall dispose of its records as directed by a court of appropriate jurisdiction.

2. Dangerous and Narcotic drugs related records

These are drugs which are likely to cause drug abuse. Hence, there are special provision for prescribing these drugs, storing and maintenance of their records.

The practitioners authorized to prescribe or dispense controlled substance shall maintain a record with the following information :

(a) name and address of patient

(b) date prescribed
(c) name, strength and amount of medication.

The information for prescribed controlled substances may be kept either in a log or on patient records provided such records or logs are made available for inspection. The information for dispensed controlled substances must be maintained in a separate log at least 8 by 11 inches in dimension. Entries must include the date dispensed, name and address of the patient, name and strength of medication, and amount dispensed.

Other persons registered to manufacture, distribute, or dispense controlled substances shall maintain a record with the following information :

(a) amount received or distributed.
(b) names, addresses and dates regarding these transactions.

Accountability Audits

Pharmacies : Accountability audits in pharmacies will be accomplished through a review of invoices, prescription files, other records required.

Medical, dental and veterinary : Accountability audits of medical, dental and veterinary practitioners will be accomplished through a review of records to be kept.

Manufacturers and distributors : Accountability audits of manufacturers and distributors (including wholesalers) will be accomplished through a review of invoices received and distributed.

Final inventory

Pharmacies : Whenever the pharmacist in charge of a pharmacy leaves his position, a complete inventory of all medication will be taken by the present and prospective pharmacist-in-charge. A copy of such inventory will be sent to the Office of Narcotics and Dangerous Drugs and another copy retained on the premises.

For the purpose of this regulation, the "pharmacist-in-charge" is a pharmacist registered with the State Board of pharmacy and who is responsible for the prescription department of the registrant.

Medical, dental and veterinary : Medical, dental and veterinary practitioners who cease legal existence or discontinue business or professional practice shall notify the Office of Narcotics and Dangerous Drugs promptly of such fact, and shall provide the office with an inventory off controlled substance on hand.

Retention of records

All records required by this Regulation must be retained for a period of at least two (2) years.

Prescriptions

Definitions : As used in this section:

(i) The term "Act" means the Narcotic and Dangerous Drugs Act.

(ii) The term "individual practitioner" means physician, dentist, veterinarian, or other individual, licensed, registered to dispense a controlled substance in the course of professional practice but does not include a pharmacist, a pharmacy, or an institutional practitioner.

(iii) The term "pharmacist" means any pharmacist licensed by the State pharmacy council to dispense controlled substances and shall include any other person (e.g. pharmacist intern) authorized by the State of Delaware to dispense controlled substances under the supervision of a pharmacist licensed by this State.

(iv) The term "prescription" means an order for medication which is dispensed to or for an ultimate user but does not include an order for medication which is dispensed for immediate administration to the ultimate user (e.g, an order to dispense a drug to a bed patient for immediate administration in a hospital is not a prescription).

(v) The terms "register" and "registered" refer to registration required by State Pharmacy Council.

(vi) Persons entitled to issue prescriptions

A prescription for a controlled substance may be issued only by an individual practitioner who is:

(a) Authorized to prescribe controlled substances by the jurisdiction in which he is licensed to practice his profession; and

(b) A verbal prescription for a controlled substance may only be communicated to a pharmacist by the prescriber. Prescriptions for controlled substances communicated by an employee or agent of the prescriber are not valid.

(c) Written prescriptions for controlled substances may be transmitted via facsimile by a practitioner or by the practitioner's authorized agent to a pharmacy only when the transmission complies with Act governing the dangerous drugs.

Purposes of Issue of Prescription

A prescription for a controlled substance to be effective, must be issued for a legitimate medical purpose by an individual practitioner acting in the usual course of his professional practice. The responsibility for proper prescribing and dispensing of controlled substances is upon the prescribing practitioner, but a corresponding responsibility rests with the pharmacist who fills the prescription. An order purporting to be a prescription not issued in the usual course of professional treatment or in legitimate and authorized research is not a prescription within the meaning and intent of the Act and the person knowingly filling such a purported prescription, as well as the person issuing it shall be subject to the penalties provided for violation of the provisions of law relating to controlled substances.

A prescription may not be issued in order for an individual practitioner to obtain controlled substances for supplying the individual practitioner for the purpose of general dispensing to patients.

A prescription may not be issued for the dispensing of narcotic drugs listed in any schedule to a narcotic drug dependent person for the purpose of continuing his dependence upon such drugs, unless otherwise authorized by law.

Manner of issuance of prescriptions

All prescriptions for controlled substances shall be dated and signed on the day when issued and shall bear the full name and address of the patient, and the name, address and registration number of the practitioner. A practitioner may sign a prescription in the same manner as he would sign a check or legal document. When an oral order is not permitted, prescriptions shall be written with ink or indelible pencil or typewriter and shall be manually signed by the practitioner. The prescriptions may be prepared by a secretary or agent for the signature of a practitioner but the prescribing practitioner is responsible where the prescription does not conform in all essential respects to the law and regulations. A corresponding liability rests upon the pharmacist who fills a prescription not prepared in the form prescribed by these regulations. Each written prescription shall have the name of the practitioner stamped, typed, or hand-printed on it, as well as the signature of the practitioner.

Persons entitled to fill prescriptions

A prescription for controlled substances may only be filled by a pharmacist acting in the usual course of his professional practice and either registered individually or employed in a registered pharmacy or by a registered institutional practitioner.

Emergency dispensing of dangerous drugs

In an emergency situation a pharmacist may dispense controlled substances listed in the Schedule upon receiving oral authorization of a prescribing individual practitioner, provided that the procedures comply with Federal law and regulation.

Expiration of prescription

Prescriptions for controlled substances in Schedules will become void unless dispensed within seven (7) days of the original date of the prescription or if the original prescriber authorizes the prescription past the seven (7) days period. Such prescriptions cannot be written nor dispensed for more than 100 dosage units or a 31 day supply whatever is the greater at one time.

Mail order prescription

Before dispensing prescriptions for controlled substances by mail, the registrant and/or the pharmacist-in-charge must assure that the prescription is valid and written by a prescriber properly registered with the Federal Government. Such verification may be made either in writing or orally.

The pharmacist must establish that the non-resident physician or dentist is properly registered to prescribe controlled substances under Federal Law. The pharmacist may keep a record which contains the name and address of the non-resident physician or dentist, his Federal registration number, and the name and address of the source of the registration data.

The pharmacist must verify the identification of the bearer of the prescription by reference to a driver's license or some other identification which contains the bearer's photograph, and must keep a record of such person.

Security and Disposal

Pharmacies and medical, dental and veterinary practitioners must store controlled substances in a burglar resistant type safe or grade steel cabinet or their equivalent. If the safe weighs less than 750 pounds, it must be bolted, cemented, or secured to the wall or floor in such a way that it cannot be readily removed. Other types of substantially construed, securely locked cabinets or drawers are acceptable provided that the room, storage area or areas shall be provided with electronic intrusion detection equipment to all sections of the said area or areas where controlled substances are stored, so as to detect any mishappening.

The Secretary may require additional security requirements if he deems it necessary as a result of excessive diversion of controlled substances.

Safes, cabinets or drawers containing Schedule II controlled substances must be kept locked at all times. They may be opened only by the practitioner or by the pharmacist-in charge or other designees, who must be licensed medical professionals.

Practitioners who store no more than 400 total dosage units of controlled substances are not required to comply with the safe or alarm requirements of the regulation. However, their controlled substances must be stored in securely locked, substantially constructed cabinets.

Report of Loss or Theft

Registrants shall notify the Office of Narcotics and Dangerous Drugs, Division of Public Health, of any theft or significant loss of any controlled substances, or of any prescription blanks, upon the discovery of such loss or theft. In addition, registrants shall complete the Federal forms regarding such loss or theft, one copy of which must be filed with the Office of Narcotics and Dangerous Drugs.

Disposal of Controlled Substances

Any registrant in possession of any controlled substances and desiring or required to dispose of such substance or substances shall contact the Office of Narcotics and Dangerous Drugs of the Division of Public Health for proper instructions regarding disposal.

Disposal of Hypodermic Syringe or Needle

Hypodermic syringes or needles shall be destroyed before disposal in such a manner as will render it impossible to adapt them for the use of narcotic drugs by subcutaneous injections.

3. Emergency Kit or Emergency Drugs related records

Each rehabilitation center, upon the advice and written approval of the facility's physician, must maintain an emergency kit or stock supply of drugs and medicines for the use of the physician in treating the emergency needs of his patient. This kit or medicine shall be stored in such a manner as to limit its access to authorized personnel, but in such a manner as to allow quick retrieval. This emergency drug supply shall be assessed only when licensed personnel are on duty.

Requirements for hospital emergency drugs or emergency drug kits or other storage method for emergency drugs are as follows:

1. Pharmacy policy and procedures shall assure the:
   (A) availability;
   (B) control; and
   (C) security;
   of emergency drug kits in the pharmacy and patient care areas.
2. Procedures shall include the following:
   (A) Determination of drugs and quantities of drugs to be included.
   (B) Labeling for expiration date.
   (C) Process for restocking the cart, kit, or box.
   (D) Security measures to prevent unauthorized access.
3. All drugs in the emergency drug kit shall be selected and approved by a committee whose membership includes, at a minimum, the following:
   (A) The facility's consultant pharmacist.
   (B) A licensed nurse.
   (C) A physician (medical doctor or doctor of osteopathy).
   (D) The facility administrator.
4. The selection process must identify drugs and quantities there of in the emergency drug kit.
5. The lists of drugs and quantities included in the emergency drug kit shall be reviewed as required periodically, but no less often than yearly.
6. Labeling as follows:
   (i) The exterior labeling of the emergency drug kit as described in this subsection shall contain, at a minimum, the following:
      (A) Drug name (trade name, generic name, or active ingredients).
      (B) Drug strength or size, if any.
      (C) Quantity included therein.
      (D) Expiration date of the kit as defined in this section.

(ii) All drugs contained in the emergency drug kit as described in this section shall be labeled, at a minimum, with the following:

(A) Drug name (trade name, generic name, or active ingredients).

(B) Drug strength or size, if applicable.

(C) Name of the manufacturer, packer, or distributor.

(D) Lot number.

(E) Expiration date : The expiration date of the emergency drug kit, as required in subsection shall be the earliest date of expiration of any of the drugs included in the kit at any time.

7. All emergency kits subject to this subsection :

(A) shall be stored in a secure area, suitable for the prevention of unauthorized access to or diversion of the drugs therein;

(B) if controlled substances, as defined in the act, are stored in such a manner as to facilitate periodic reconciliation by the facility nursing staff, that reconciliation shall be recorded in an appropriate manner as determined by the committee described under this section; and

(C) all controlled substances contained in emergency drug kits shall remain the property of the supplying pharmacy and as such shall be included in the pharmacy's biennial inventory.

8. The nurse responsible for removing drugs from an emergency drug kit shall record, in a manner designated, with the following minimum information :

(A) Name of the patient.

(B) Name of the drug.

(C) Strength of the drug.

(D) Quantity removed.

(E) Date of removal.

(F) Time of removal.

(j) Removal of a controlled substance in Schedule II pursuant to an oral authorization from a practitioner shall be documented.

9. Whenever an emergency kit is opened, for any reason, the supplying pharmacy shall be notified in a timely manner, and the pharmacy shall restock, if necessary, and reseal the kit promptly so as to prevent risk of harm to the facility in emergency situation.

4. Maintenance of Records for Ward Stock Medicines

These are the medicines, kept in the ward for the use of in-patients.

(i) The male or female nurses send the requirements on requisition form to the central medical store. This form is duly signed by the medical officer in charge of the concerning ward.

(ii) The supply is received and entered in the register for record.

(iii) The drug is issued for the patient use (recorded in the medical file of the patient) and recorded in the daily consumption.

(iv) This helps in handing over the charge to the next person taking the charge.

13
Chapter

Applications of Computers in Pharmacy

It is well known that information processing and computers have penetrated all aspects of modern human life. The medical profession has been affected perhaps more than others, taking advantage of advanced IT technology with high networking and integration capabilities and quality image display support. Of course, computers will never replace doctor patient relationships in most healthcare areas. However, computers have been widely adopted in different stages of medical care to achieve effective information collection, precise data analysis, and to aid in forming final treatment decisions.

In this chapter, some of the Hospital/Hospital related applications of computers are illustrated.

1. Role of Computers in Registration Process and Medical Record Keeping

Record keeping is poor in most of the Government hospitals in India. The number of patients is so large that it becomes almost impossible to keep a track. There are long queues on the registration counters and files are traceable with great difficulty for follow up consultation. There are heaps of files stacked in record rooms which are very hard to retrieve. Valuable data about patients and different diagnostic features stored in patient files becomes untraceable because of huge number of files.

The condition becomes pitiable for patients seen in emergency condition where the knowledge of previous health and disease status is required and available time is short. In addition, there are problems of storage space, missing pages of records due to mishandling and also illegibility. The whole problem can be solved if the whole registration process and medical record keeping are computerized. The initial effort and investement may be discouraging but it shall prove to be an asset in the long term. The system is quick and efficient, reduces waiting time and improves retrievability.

In most of the big sized hospitals in India, for example , Escort, Apollo Hospitals, there is a main centralized computer with terminals available at all registration counters and other work place. Each patient, who comes for consultation is given a unique registration number. Even if a patient is seen in more than one departmental clinic, the same number shall suffice and multiplicity of clinic number may be avoided. Details of age, address, sex, marital status and other diagnostic data are recorded. The complete computerized patient registration record is available to each clinic dealing with the patient from a single data base.

In other hospitals, unique 'pass words' are provided to the users. Therefore, the user is identified by the computer and recorded. This avoids the unauthorized use to maintain secrecy.

To fulfill these requirements, one would need a sophisticated/ advanced computer, a large number of terminals, display units and printers, memory storage discs and tapes. Above all, there is need of expert or technically sound manpower to run the computerized system.

A master index of all patients is created in the central registration department (CRD). Whenever a patient reports to the out-patient department for follow up check up or in emergency department, the master index is searched to check up his previous medical records. Even if the previous registration number is not known, the search from the master index can be made easily using the patient's name, place of residence or disease state, etc.

It is important to add the recent/newer data in the patient file regarding revisits, admissions, discharges, transfers between wards, interspeciality consultations and added problems and disease complications. This continuous monitoring is essential for up to date knowledge about the patient as well as for statutory on hospital statistics regarding total attendance, admissions, bed occupancy and mortality. Break up patient statistics are done according to age, sex, occupation and consultancy obtained. For example, one can easily obtain history of rheumatic cases between a particular age group over particular period of time.

2. Role of Computers in medical research

In medical research, computers have two kinds of applications :

(i) Computerized diagnostic equipments

(ii) Data collection

The first use is beyond the realms of this article except to say that most of the modern equipments, be it small or big, has built in computer system. Some common examples are : MRI, computerized spirometers, blood chemistry and gas analyzer, ultra sound scanners and CT scanners. All these equipments are used for diagnostic purposes and data/ diagnostic features are automatically displayed on computer screen during examination. These data/images from CT scans, ultrasounds and X-rays can be viewed on the computer anywhere in the world.

The second application or major use relates to research planning, data collection, data analysis and statistics. The computer software may varies depending on individual needs. For example, the physiologist may require computer for creating mathematical models or for analysis of biological signal, records, graphs and images. The computer analysis of complex data is not very fast, simple and reliable but also mandatory when manual calculations become impractical.

3. Role of Computers in Drug Information System

The Drug Information System (DIS) is a computer-based system where information on all prescription drugs dispensed will be gathered and securely stored electronically linked to all health care sites, such as:

- pharmacies
- physicians' offices
- health centres
- addiction centres
- hospital pharmacies
- Emergency Departments

accessible to authorized health care professionals, including physicians and pharmacists intended to support the delivery of health care to patients .

The Drug Information System will :

- reduce the potential for harmful drug interactions, prescription errors, and adverse drug reactions
- make it easier for pharmacists to report adverse drug reactions
- help pharmacists to counsel patients about their medications
- promote better patient care by enhancing the partnership between physicians and pharmacists

- eliminate the need to repeat your medication history at each visit to your physician or pharmacist

3. Role of Computers in Drug Inventory Control

Drug control procedure is necessary to prevent the purchasing in excess and to avoid the out of stock situation which may be dangerous in emergency cases. Inventory control is still done manually in most of the general hospital as well as in retail pharmacy in India. It needs more staff and more time to check the stock situation at regular intervals by counting the number of items. One has check manually the batch number and date of expiry. But some private hospital and organized retail pharmacy have the computerized system for the inventory control. It is more accurate, time saving and economical. In the computerized system, each drug is allotted code number. Thus the quantity of each drug is entered code wise received from the supplier and issued to various department. The batch number, date of expiry and supplier name are also recorded. Minimum stock balance of every drug is marked. It is the drug quantity which must be present to avoid the out of stock situation. When minimum stock situation is reached, computer signals for placing the order of that particular drug.

The user pharamacist can collect the entire information about a drug viz; stock position, shelf life, batch number, current consumption rate, buffer stock to be maintained, expiry date, mode of purchase, sources approved, indication for the submission of the fresh indent, issuing details and all other related information about the drug which shall be flashed on the screen.

4. Role of computers in Monitoring Drug Utilization Trends

The latest Visual CE application is being used to track drug utilization trends within the hospital. The Pharmacy department conducts studies to identify changes in medication usage that can improve the quality of patient care or provide more cost-effective treatment. Typically, pharmacists will visit patients taking a particular medicine, review their charts, and gather all necessary information to assess whether utilization of the medicine is appropriate. The application captures information such as why a particular medication was prescribed, the dosage, the patient's age and physical condition, and how the patient responded to the therapy.

At the end of the day, the pharmacist synchronizes the medication data to the Pharmacy department's central system at the same time as their consulting records. A medication usage database is aggregated over time, and provides the ability to generate reports by patient demographics and medical conditions. Lawton or his staff present their findings in the hospital's medical committee meetings, and recommend changes in the utilization of the medication when appropriate.

5. Role of Computers in Adverse Drug Reaction Reporting

Because of a rapid increase in the list of newer drugs launched in the market in the last few decades; adverse drug reaction monitoring of these drugs has assumed prime importance. Since India is a country, which caters to the maximum number of human population for the final assessment of drug safety as a part of post marketing surveillance studies, it becomes necessary to report any untoward reaction of any pharmaceutical product.

The drugs, which are marketed in India, are pretested on very small population groups of European countries in an optimal environment and the data about the drug safety collected from that population could not be applied straight in our population because of the climactic and corporal differences. The Adverse Drug Reactions (ADRs) are the fourth to sixth leading cause of death among hospitalised patients and it occurs in 0.3 per cent to 7 per cent of all hospital admissions. The incidence of serious ADRs is 6.7 per cent and 30 per cent to 60 per cent of these ADRs are preventable.

Adverse drug reaction may be due to drug-drug interaction, allergy, averse effects, etc. For reporting purposes, FDA categorises serious adverse event (event related to drug or devices) as one in which "the patient outcome is death, life-threatening (real risk of dying), hospitalisation (initial or prolonged), disability (significant, persistent, or permanent), congenital anomaly, or required intervention to prevent permanent impairment or damage." For observing drug-drug reaction, the computer software programme MEDIPHOR can be used which increases the efficiency of clinical services provided by the hospital pharmacist.

The computerised drug order entry is screened here for events related to adverse drug reaction and a detailed investigation is done if any clue is found.

- Medication order screening
- Abrupt medication discontinuation.

- Abrupt dosage reduction.
- Orders for tracer substances.
- Orders for special tests or serum drug concentrations.
- Orders for high risk drugs, which are likely to cause ADRs are screened and their use is monitored

Examples of high risk drugs are aminoglycosides, amphotericin, antineoplastics, corticosteroids, digoxin, heparin, lidocaine, phenytoin, theophylline, thrombolytic agents, and Warfarin.

6. Role of Computers in Pharmacokinetics

'NONLIN' is a programme which can predict the Pharmacokinetic parameters like absorption, distribution, bioavailability, rate of excretion. From this programme, further dose can be adjusted to maintain the effective drug concentration in blood.

7. Role of Computers in Emergency Situation

Decrease errors in care by allowing emergency providers and other practitioners to quickly access the patient's complete records from anywhere in the world. In emergency, the complete diagnostic features can be send to other advanced country for expert comments.

8. Role of Computers in Finance control in Hospitals

The basic ledger system deals with the day-to-day purchases that the hospital needs to keep going on a day to day basis. It covers everything that is bought by the hospital and accounts for their purchase and their use by a particular department. All departments have budgets and these are then managed by the computer system. The finance system also manages the payroll needs of the hospital. This is the basis by which health authority pays the salary of each individual. Computers are used for billing process of patient.

14
Chapter

Nomenclature and Uses of Surgical and Hospital Equipments

Surgical instruments : Various types of instruments are used in surgical operation and it is difficult to mention all. The hospital pharmacists must be familiar with some instruments which are illustrated here.

HAEMOSTATIC FORCEPS

The name haemostatic forceps is more accurate than artery forceps because these forceps are used for both arteries and veins. However, the term artery forceps is very commonly used.

There are four common varieties :

1. **Ordinary (Spencer Wells' forceps) :** These may be curved or straight and are used to catch or hold ordinary bleeding vessels. The transverse serrations on the blades prevent slipping of the tissues held between them (Fig. 14.1).

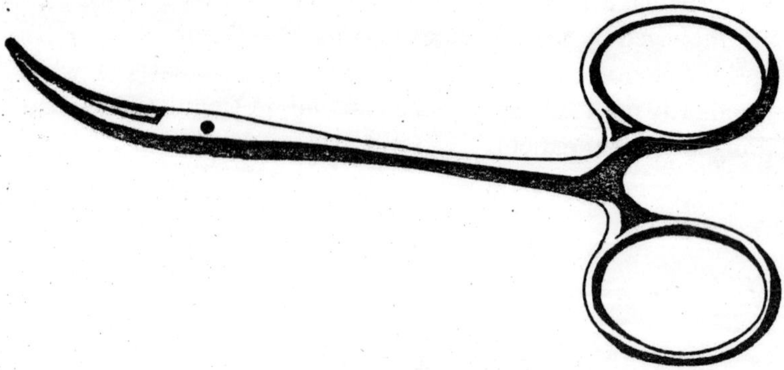

Fig. 14.1. Ordinary (Spencer Wells') attery forceps (curves).

2. **Kocher's artery forceps :** This forceps differs from an ordinary artery forceps in that it has a tooth at the tip of the blades. It is, therefore, used to hold bleeding vessel in a tough/fibrous background or vessels having a tendency to retract (Fig. 14.2).

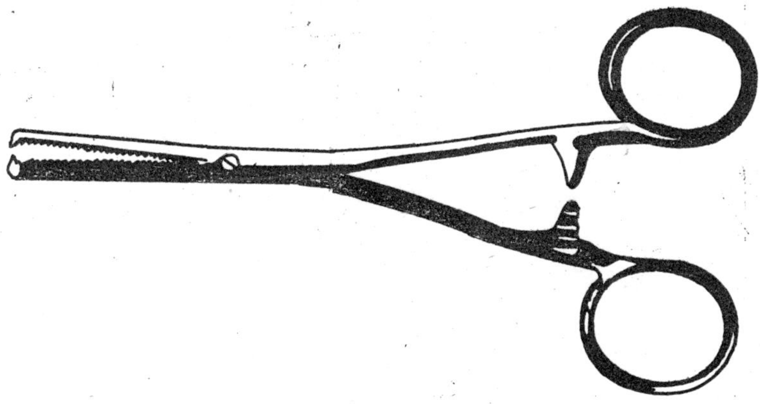

Fig. 14.2. Kocher's artery forceps (straight).

3. **Lane's artery forceps :** This is a long instrument. The handles of the instrument are long and its blades are very short. Each blade has transverse serration and tooth at the tip. It is usually used to catch bleeding periosteal vessels (Fig. 14.3).

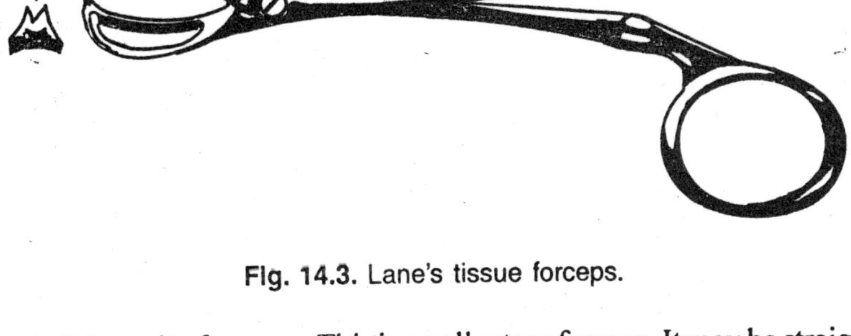

Fig. 14.3. Lane's tissue forceps.

4. **Mosquito forceps :** This is small artery forceps. It may be straight or curved. It is used to catch small bleeding vessels (Fig. 14.4).

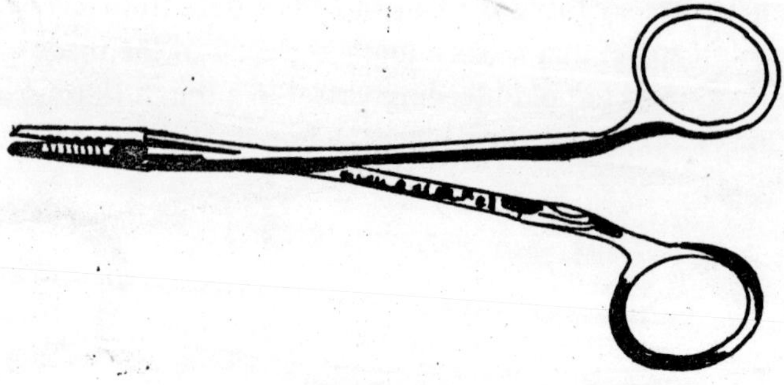

Fig. 14.4. Mosquito forceps (straight).

TISSUE FORCEPS

These forceps are used to hold tissues – either tissues to be left or tissues to be excised. The commonly used varieties are :

1. **Allis tissue forceps :** It is delicate and short (Fig. 14.5). The teeth on the blades are delicate to make this instrument useful for holding sensitive tissues, e.g. soft muscles, intestine, etc.

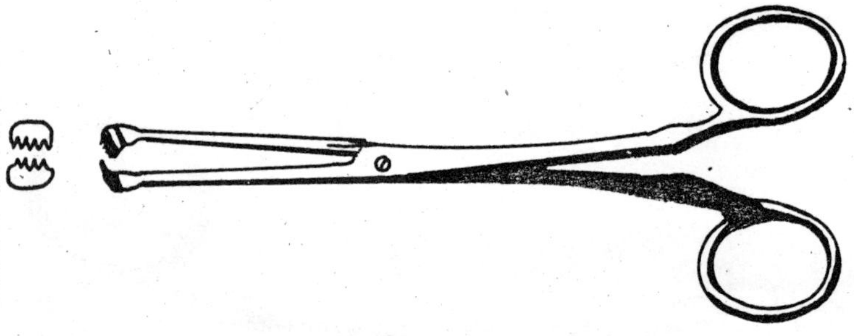

Fig. 14.5. Allis' tissue forceps.

2. **Babcock's tissue forceps :** The blades are fenestrated and there is no teeth on the blades. They are designed to hold the intestines (Fig. 14.6).
3. **Rutherford Morison's tissue forceps :** This is originally used to hold the peritoneum (hence called peritoneum forceps). Its uses are the same as Allis tissue forceps but as its teeth are sharp, the forceps should be on the intestines (Fig. 14.7).

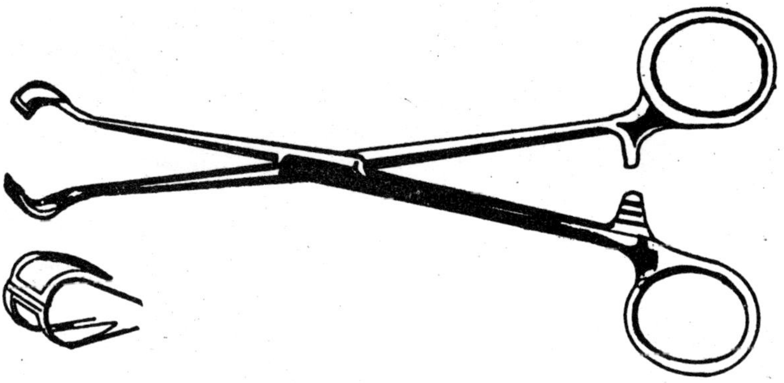

Fig. 14.6. Babcock's tissue forceps.

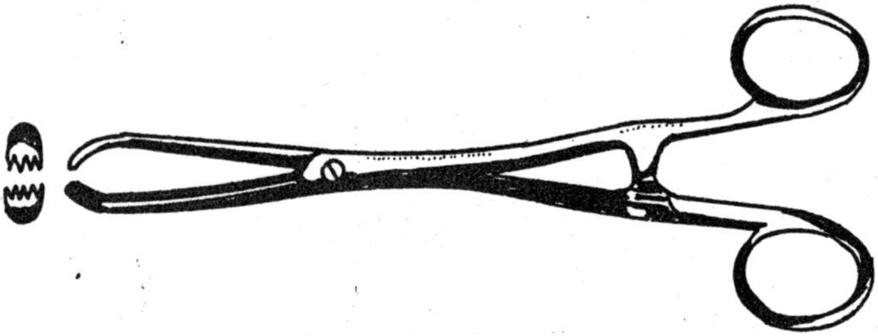

Fig. 14.7. Rutherford Morison's tissue forceps.

DISSECTING FORCEPS

These may be plain or toothed. These are used to hold the tissues during the process of dissection or suturing (Fig. 14.8).

DRESSING FORCEPS

This is a short instrument and the tips of the blades are spoon shaped

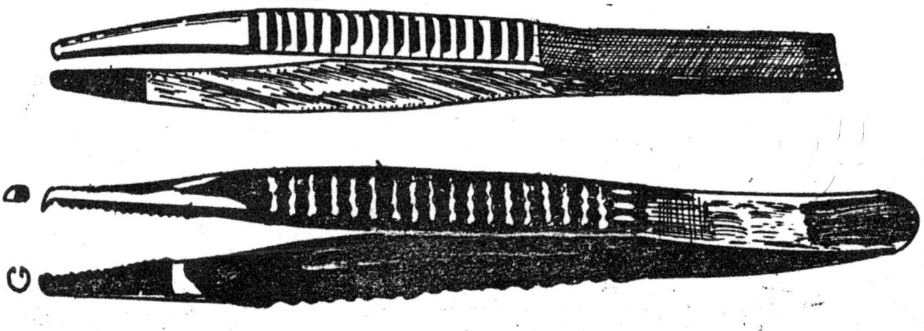

Fig. 14.8. Dissecting forceps.

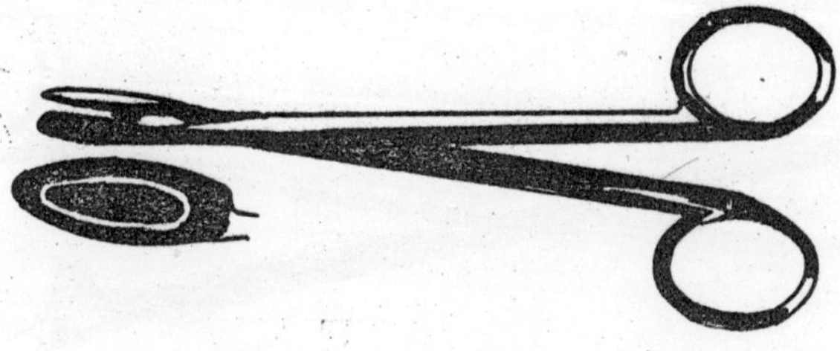

Fig. 14.9. Dissecting forceps.

having transverse serration and a central groove. There are no catches on the handles. It is used to hold a while dressing wounds (Fig. 14.9).

CHEATLE'S FORCEPS

It is stout and long instrument. It is used to take out the surgical instruments from sterilizer and to hand over to the surgeons (Fig. 14.10).

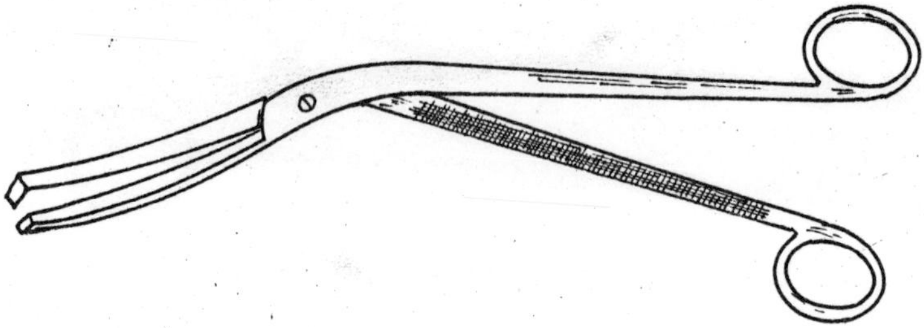

Fig. 14.10. Cheatle's forceps.

MOYNIHAN'S TETRA FORCEPS

There are four teeth in the forceps, two on each blade. It is used to fix the tetra towels to the skin flap on either side of an incision to prevent entry of bacteria from the skin surface (Fig. 14.11).

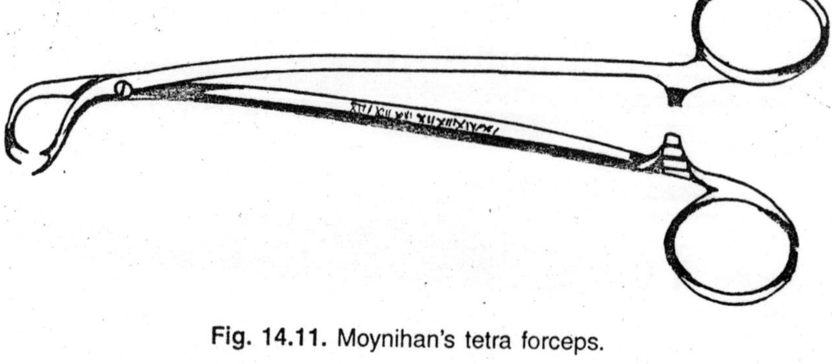

Fig. 14.11. Moynihan's tetra forceps.

BONE CUTTING FORCEPS

These forceps are used to cut small and weaker bones, e.g. phalanges and metacarpals. Bigger bones are cut with saw (Fig. 14.12).

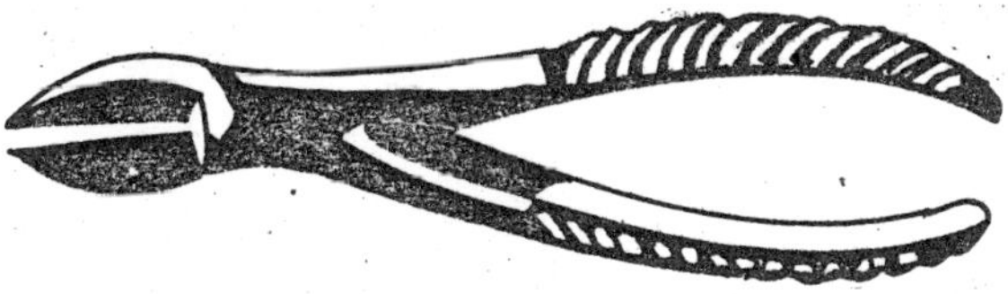

Fig. 14.12. Bone cutting forceps.

SCISSORS

These may be straight or curved, sharp or blunt pointed (Fig. 14.13).

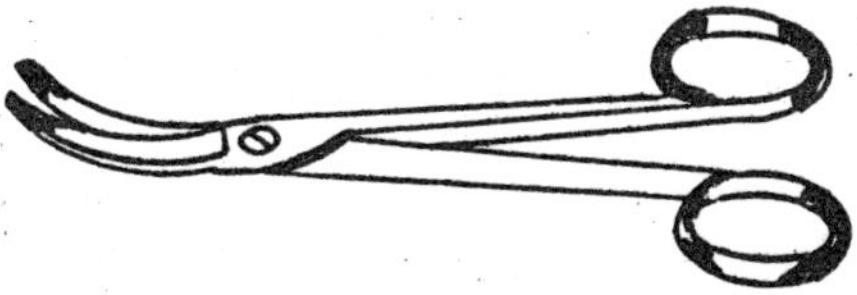

Fig. 14.13. Scissor.

SCALPEL

It is used to make incision in the skin. Stiles's type is shown (Fig. 14.14).

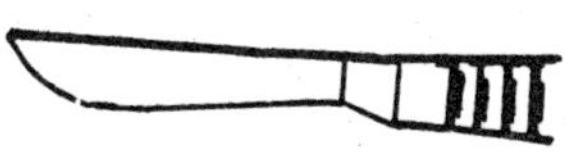

Fig. 14.14. Scalpel.

BARD-PARKER KNIFE

Like the safety razor, the blades are renewed when blunt. The blades are of various size and shapes but the principle of attaching them to the appropriate handle is standardised (Fig. 14.15).

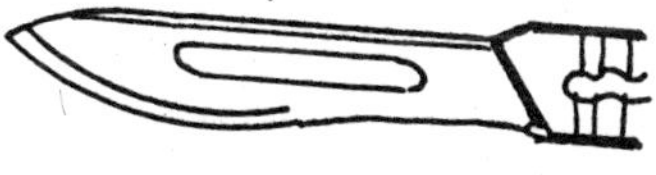

Fig. 14.15. Bard-Parked knife.

ABSCESS KNIFE

It is a convenient instrument for opening abscesses by transfixion (Fig. 14.16).

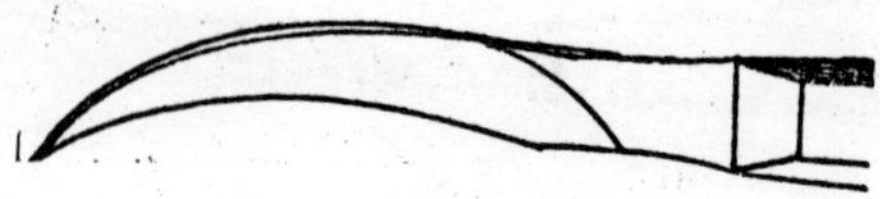

Fig. 14.16. Abscess knife.

AMPUTATION KNIFE

It is used to cut all soft tissues, down to the periosteum in amputation (Fig. 14.17).

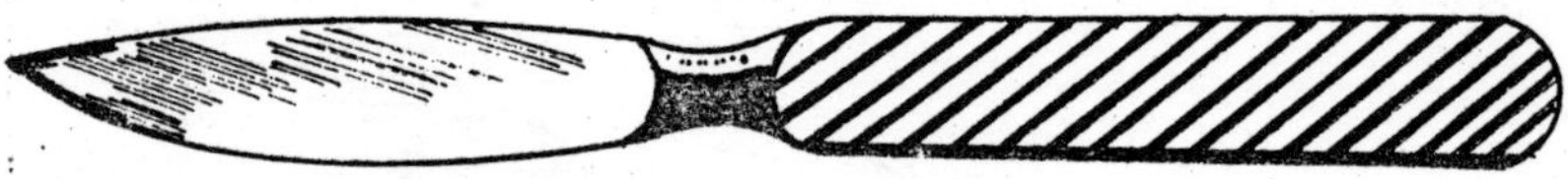

Fig. 14.17. Amputation knife.

VOLKMANN'S SPOON

It is used as scoop to scrape sinus, fistula and chronic ulcers and as spoon to collect contents from inside a cavity or to put some antiseptic powder into a cavity or wound (Fig. 14.18).

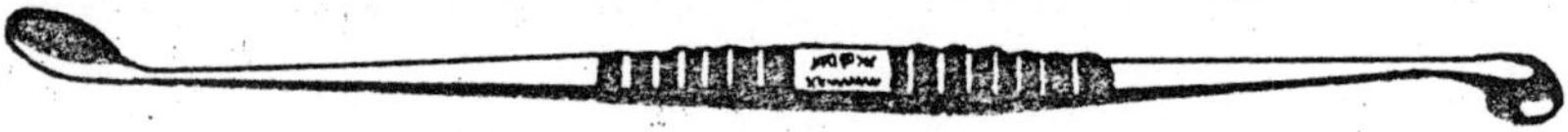

Fig. 14.18. Volkmann's spoon (scoop).

SWAB HOLDER

This is a long instrument with the blades expanded at their ends where there are transverse serrations and a central fenestration. It is used to hold a swab in order to cleanse the field of operation in the depth (Fig. 14.19).

NEEDLES

Needles are used for suturing the tissues and may be straight or curved. Curvature may be half circle, 3/8th or 5/8th of a circle. In general, the straight needles are used while working on the surface and the curved needles at the depth. According to the cross section, a needle may be (a) round, (b) triangular, (c) flat. While differentiating between a round bodied and triangular cutting needle–the cross section towards the tip

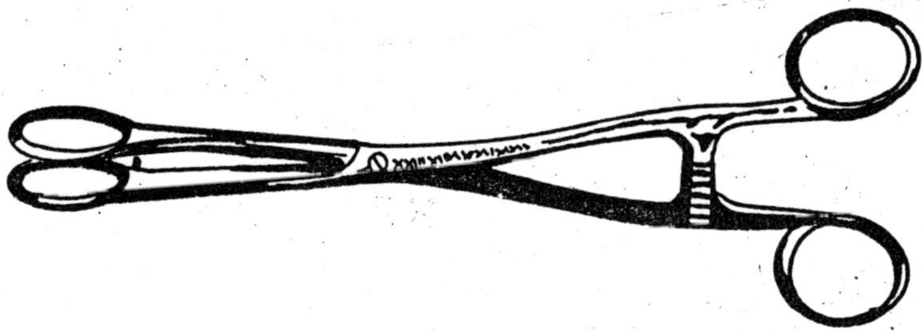

Fig. 14.19. Swab holder.

should be considered since all these needles are round bodied towards eye (Fig. 14.20).

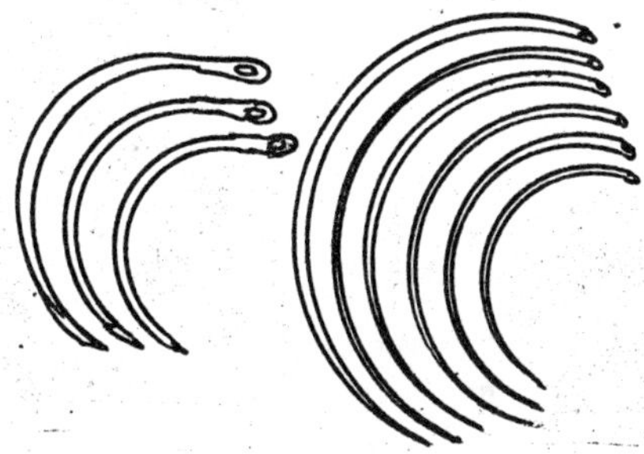

Fig. 7.20. Surgical needles.

NEEDLE HOLDER

This may be straight or curved. It is used to hold the needle while suturing. The straight needle holders are used on the surface and the curved holders are conveniently used in the depth (Fig. 14.21).

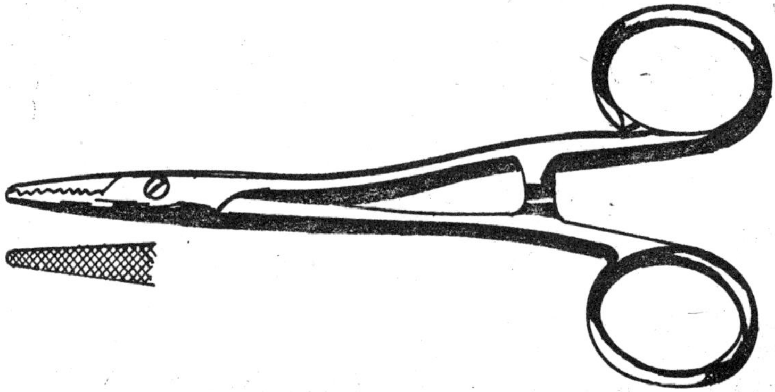

Fig. 14.21. Needle holder.

TONGUE DEPRESSOR

It is used for depressing the tongue to examine the tonsils and posterior wall of the pharynx (Fig. 14.22).

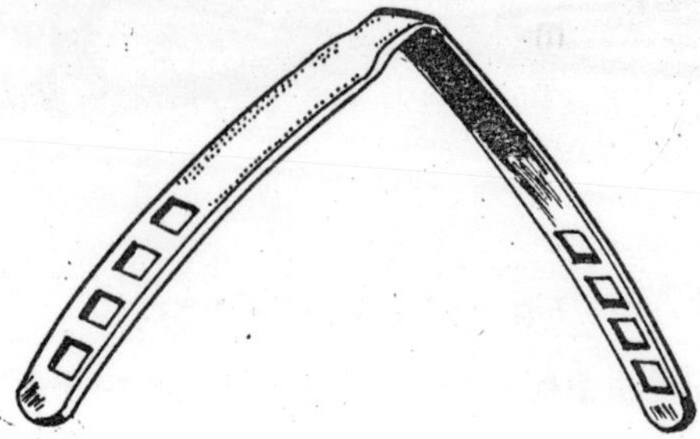

Fig. 14.22. Tongue depresser.

TOWEL CLIP

1. **The pinchter type :** It is used to hold the corners of the drapping sheets at operation (Fig. 14.23).

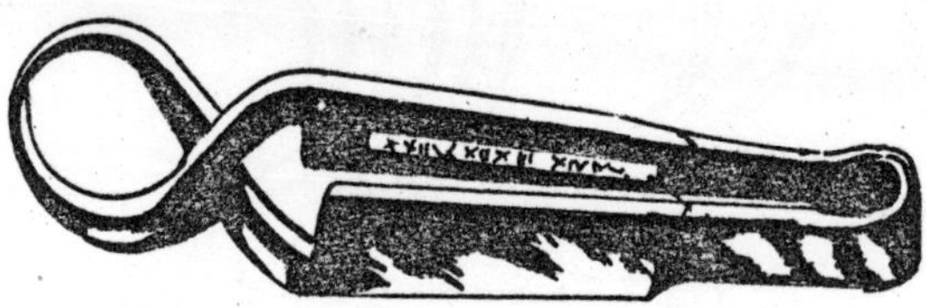

Fig. 14.23. Towel clip (pinchter type).

2. **The forcep type :** It is used as a tongue holding forceps (Fig. 14.24).

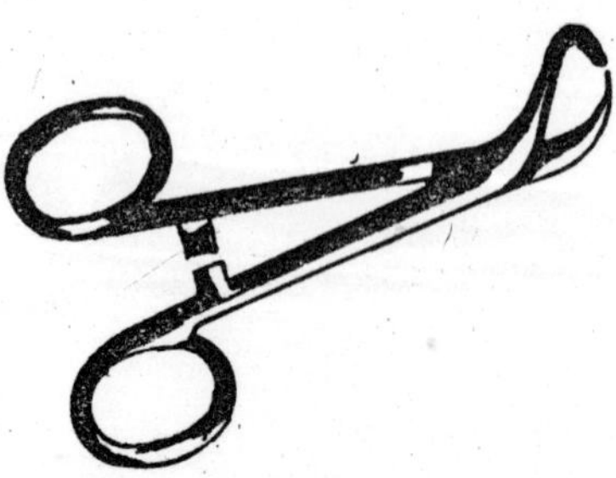

Fig. 14.24. Towel clip (forcep type).

SYRINGES

These are used to administer drug by various parenteral routes, e.g. subcutaneous, intravenous and intramuscular. The pioneer syringe consists of needle attachment accommodating all needle sizes. The tuberculin syringe is a small syringe not exceeding 1 ml capacity and graduated 0.1 to 0.01 ml divisions. The hypodermic syringe is usually 2 to 50 ml capacity. There are larger piston syringes ranging up to 200 ml for transfusion and irrigation purposes. Insulin syringes have unit graduation (40 or 100 units) rather than volume graduations.

HOSPITAL EQUIPMENTS

Various type of equipments are used depending on specialization but there are some essential equipments listed below which must be installed in all general hospitals.

1. **X-ray machine :** It is used to observe the abnormalities present inside.
2. **ECG machine :** It takes the electroradiogram to observe the proper functioning of heart. It is an essential equipment of cardio-vascular unit. In the heart hospital, automatic analysers are attached with ECG machine which give the direct interpretation.
3. **B.P. apparatus :** Either sphygmomanometer or electronic machine is used to measure the blood pressure.
4. **Glucometer :** Compact machine, called glucometer, is available in many hospitals which measures the blood sugar in a quick time and stores the previous result in memory.
5. **Bone densitometer :** It is used to measure bone mass. Bone mass, simply put, is the weight of the skeleton, overall or in specific region.
6. **Laryngosopes :** It is used to obtain a view of vocal cords and glottis which is the space between the cords.
7. **Resuscitator :** It is a device using positive pressure to inflate the lungs of an unconscious person who is not breathing.
8. **Nebulizer :** It changes asthma medication from a liquid to a mist, so that it can be more easily inhaled into the lungs.

Specialized big sized hospitals also contain the following equipments :

1. **CT scanner :** It is used to perform the morphological analysis of internal organs.
2. **Ultrasound sonography equipment :** It is helpful to take the internal picture which is specially helpful to know the reasons of repeated abortion, foetal conditions and abnormalities.
3. **Magnetic resonance imaging (MRI) :** It is an aid to neurosurgery for diagnosis of complicated cases, e.g. nerve lesions, tumors, etc.

15

Chapter

Surgical Dressings

Surgical dressing is a term to a wide range of materials used for dressing of wounds. They are used as coverings, absorbents, protectives or supports for injured or diseased tissues. Dressings may be classified as :

1. Primary Wound Dressings

These are dressings, directly placed on a wound surface and are usually reinforced by materials of various types to absorb the wound secretion.

Gauze compresses of suitable mesh and thickness are widely used as primary wound dressings but they have the drawback of adherence to the wound surface. To minimize this difficulty, various types of dressings are designed to avoid the pain, caused when dressing is removed from the wound surface.

Petrolatum-impregnated gauze has been widely used for this purpose. It is hydrophobic in nature and it does not adhere to the wound surface. Gauze, knitted from regenerated cellulose and impregnated with hydrophobic oil in water emulsion, is also used asx it has extremely low degree of adherence to all types of wounds.

2. Absorbent

Surgical Cotton

Surgical cotton is the basic surgical absorbent. The bolls (fruits) contains numerous seeds with cotton fibres. Each of these fibre is a minute, hair like tube. It is flattened and twisted. The raw cotton fibre, after the seeds have been removed by gin, is mechanically cleaned of dirt and compressed into balls of various size. This form is called *non-absorbent cotton*. It is a non-absorbent due to presence of a sticky substance. It is used for padding, covering of unbroken surfaces and as cotton plugs in the bacteriological laboratory.

Adsorbent cotton is prepared from the raw cotton fibre by a series of processes which remove the natural waxes, all foreign substances and make the fibres absorbent. Fatty matter is removed by boiling the raw cotton with caustic alkali under pressure. By the treatment, fats are saponified and cellulose of hair is unaffected. The fibres are bleached with bleaching powder. They are treated with dilute acid and then washed thoroughly with water to remove all soluble matter. The product is then dried and processed to obtain roll cotton.

Besides familiar roll form, purified cotton may be obtained in the form of cotton balls.

Cotton balls can be prepared by hand or by special machines. Machine made balls are firm, compact and uniform in size, shape and weight.

The large size balls are made for obstetrical uses in the delivery room. The medium size cotton ball is particularly useful for applying antisepties or medication locally and the small cotton ball is often used for skin cleaning before hypodermic or intravenous injections.

Tests

(a) The fibres become violet on treatment with zinc chloride solution.
(b) The fibres are soluble in 66% sulphuric acid and they are insoluble in 1.25 M NaOH solution.
(c) To 0.1 g of cotton, add 10 ml of zinc chloride solution, heat to 40° and allow to stand for 2.5 hours with occasional shaking. The fibres do not dissolve.

Standards

British pharmacopoeia has recommended the following standards for absorbent cotton :

(a) When examined under microscope, each fibre is seen to consist of single cell up to about 4 cm long and 40 mm wide, in the form of a flattened tube with thick and rounded walls and often twisted, only occasional isolated fibres may be present.
(b) *Absorbency* : Absorbency indicates the absorbing capacity and represents in terms of sinking time and water holding capacity. The sinking time is not more than 10 seconds and the water holding

capacity is not more than 23.0 g^{-1} (Appendix xx, L-1, method-1 and Appendix xx, L-2 in B.P.).

(c) *Acidity or alkalinity* : To 15 g absorbent cotton, add 150 ml of water, macerate for 2 hours in closed vessel, decant the liquid, carefully squeezing out the residual liquid with a glass rod and mix. Filter it and to 25 ml of the filtered extract, add 0.1 ml of dilute phenolphthalein solution, to another 25 ml, add 0.05 ml of methyl orange solution. Neither solution shows a pink colour.

(d) *Water soluble substances* : Boil 5 g with 500 ml of water for 30 minutes and replace the water lost by evaporation. Decant the liquid into a beaker, squeeze the residual liquid from material carefully with a glass rod, mix the liquid and filter the extract whilst hot. Evaporate 400 ml and dry the residue to constant at 100° to 105°. It should not be more than 0.50% of the total weight.

(e) *Ether soluble substances* : Extract 5 g with ether in a Soxhlet apparatus for 4 hours. Evaporate the ether extract and dry the residue at 100° to 105°, unless otherwise specified in the monograph. It should not be 0.5% of the total weight.

Surgical gauzes : The function of surgical gauze is to provide an absorbent material of sufficient tensile strength for surgical dressing. For making surgical gauze, the raw cotton fibre is mechanically cleaned, spun or twisted into a thread and the thread, in turn, woven into an open-mesh cloth. The cloths is grey in appearance and non-absorbent. It is bleached white and rendered absorbent by much the same processes as used in the preparation of surgical cotton.

Gauze is classified according to its mesh or number of threads per inch. Some types of surgical dressings require a close-meshed gauze for extra strength and greater protection while primary wound dressing require softer and absorbent gauzes of more open structure.

Standards

Surgical gauze is checked for the following standards :

1. (i) Yarn number
   (ii) Thread per stated length
   (iii) Weight per unit area
   (iv) Minimum breaking load
2. *Absorbancy* : Its sinking time should not be more than 10 seconds (see absorbent cotton).

3. Acidity or alkalinity : It is checked in the same way as absorbent cotton (see absorbent cotton). Neither solution shows a pink colour.

3. Bandages

The function of bandages is to hold dressing in place to provide pressure or support. They may be inelastic, elastic or become rigid after shaping for immobilization. Various types of bandages, common in use, are listed here :

(i) *Common gauze roller bandage* : It is prepared from 'Absorbent Gauze' in various width and length. Each bandage is one continuous piece, tightly rolled and free from loose threads and ravelling.

(ii) *Muslin bandage rolls* : They are made of close mesh non-absorbent gauze. They are supplied in the same width as the regular gauze bandage. Muslin bandages are strong and are used wherever normal gauze bandage do not provide sufficient strength or support. They are frequently used to hold splints or bulky compression dressings in place.

(iii) *Crepe bandages* : It has elasticity which is due to special weave that allows it to stretch to practically twice its length even after repeated laundering. The elasticity of crepe bandages make it suitable for bandaging varicose veins, sprains, etc. because it conforms closely to the skin for joint surfaces and also allows limited motion and stretches in case of swelling so that circulation is not impaired.

(iv) *Woven elastic bandage* : It is made of heavy elastic webbing containing rubber threads. Good support and pressure are provided by this type of rubber elastic bandage.

(v) *Orthopedic bandages* : They are used to provide immobilization and support in treatment of broken bones and in certain condition of bones and joints. Plaster of Paris-impregnated gauze has been the standard for this purpose. Plaster of Paris bandages are available in wide variety of sizes.

(vi) *Stockinette bandage* : They are made of stockinette material knitted or woven in tubular form. Surgical stockinette is unbleached. It is soft and stretch readily to conform comfortably to the arm, leg or body. It is used to cover the skin prior to the application of a Plaster of Paris.

4. Adhesive Plasters

The following adhesive plasters are in common practice :

(i) Belladonna and capsicum plaster
(ii) Capsicum plaster
(iii) Zinc oxide plaster

These are pressure sensitive or self-adhesive. The adhesive action is due to the presence of rubber based adhesives or acrylate adhesives. Acrylate adhesives on a non-woven or fabric backing have been widely used in a surgical dressing application, where reduced trauma is required as in operative procedures. Rubber based adhesives are used on cloth or plastic backing. They arc used principally where heavy support and superior adhesion are required.

Acrylate adhesives are a unipolymeric system and eliminate the use of a large number of component as in rubber-based adhesives. Rubber based adhesives are composed of an elastomer (pale rubber or synthetic elastomers made from polymers of isobutylene, alkyl acrylate and similar materials), resin or modified resin, antioxidant. plasticizers (naphthaline), fillers (kieselguhr) and colouring agents to give the desired tint or whiteness.

5. Protectives

They are various impermeable materials, used adjunctively with other dressing component to prevent the loss of moisture or heat from a wound site or to protect clothing from wound exudate.

Plastic sheet and waxed or plastic coated paper are used as protectives to prevent escape of moisture or heat from dressing or compress and to protect clothing. Rubber coated cloth, which is water proof and flexible, is used as a covering for bedding.

Film dressing, used as protective, is a new concept in which acrylate adhesive coated on a transparent, moisture, vapour permeable plastic film, is applied directly on a wound surface. This type of dressing system protects the wound site because it is impervious to liquid water and bacteria but allow the passage of moisture vapour from the wound site.

HOSPITAL SUPPLY

Intravenous (I.V.) Transfusion Set

It is used to deliver fluid intravenously. They are sterilized, pyrogen free and disposable sets.

It consists of three basic units :

(i) Needle or intravenous catheter
(ii) Administration set
(iii) Container of liquid

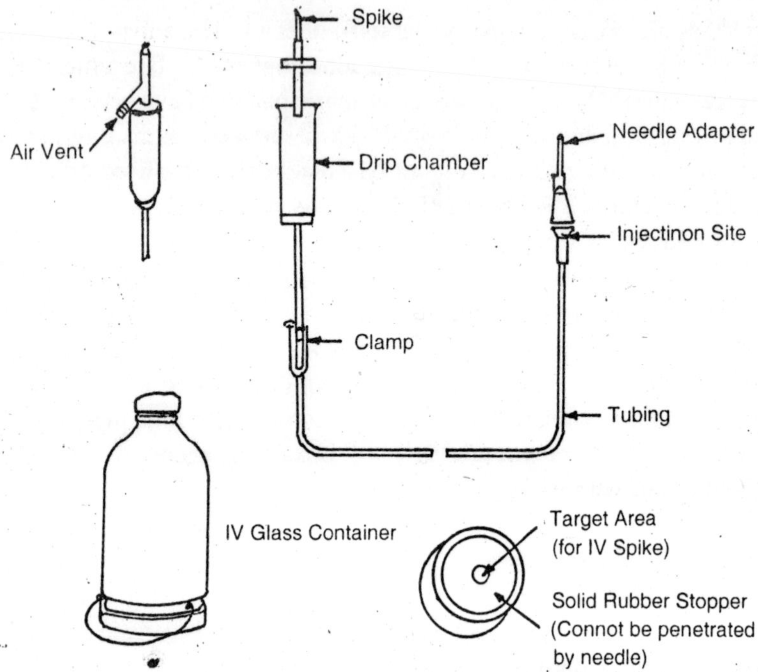

Fig. 15.1. Basic component for I.V. administration set.

Administration set includes a plastic spike or pierce the rubber closure or plastic seal on the I.V. container, a drip chamber to trap air and permit adjustment of flow rate and a length (150-450 cm) a poly-vinyl chloride tubing terminating in gum rubber injection port. At the tip of the port, rigid needle or atheter adapter is fixed. As adjustable clamp (screw or roller type) on the tubing pinches the tubing to regulate flow. Since the gum-rubber port is self-sealing, additional medication can be added to the I.V. system at these ports of entry. I.V. container is made of glass or polyvinyl chloride (flexible type). The container has no air tubes and requires air-inlet filters designed as part of the administration set.

Catheters

Catheters are used to collect the urine from unconscious patient or urinal are inadequate. Various type of catheters are available in the market.

A flexible soft rubber catheter (Fig. 15.2) consists of small rubber tubes with a closed solid tip. At one end, there is funnel-shaped opening for attachment of catheter to a glass junction or another tube leading to a collection unit. At the inserted end, wide opening is present through which urine flows to the collection unit. This type of catheter is called straight catheter.

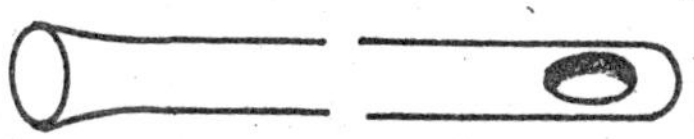

Fig. 15.2. Rubber catheter.

The indwelling retention or Foley catheter (Fig. 15.3) is designed to remain in the urethra for long periods of time. Balloon is present at the insertion end to secure the catheter tip in the patient's bladder to keep it away from slipping or being pulled out. There are two channels which run from insertion tip to the end of the Foley catheter – one for the passing of urine and other for injection of sterilized water which inflates the balloon.

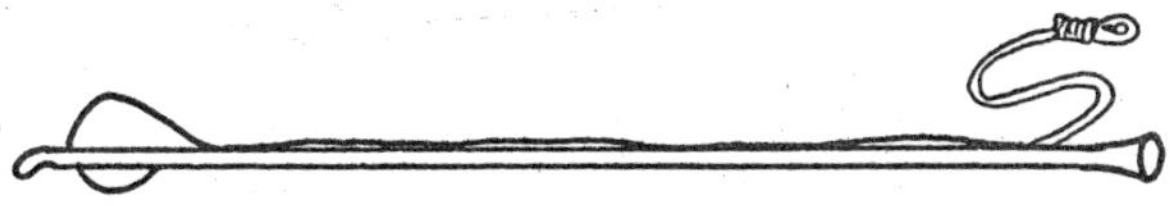

Fig. 15.3. Catheter, Foley's urethra into the bladder.

Metallic catheters are also available separately for male and female. The male catheters (Fig. 15.4) are curved because the male urethra is curved along its length. The two eyes of the catheter are not located at the level since this wound make the catheter weak at the spot. The two rings on the handle of the catheter are meant for attachment of threads

Fig. 15.4. Male metallic catheter.

that are used to fix the catheter in position. The other end of the threads is tied to the thigh of the patient on either side.

Female metallic catheter (Fig. 15.5) is comparatively short and straight because the urethra is short in length and straight. There are multiple holes at the tip because some of these may get blocked.

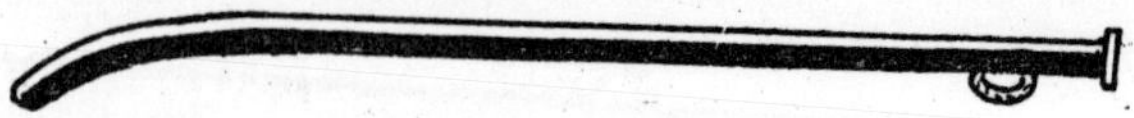

Fig. 15.5. Female metallic catheter.

Ryles tube (rubber) : It is used for sucking and feeding purposes.

Stomach tube : It is a small plastic tube placed through the nose into the stomach. The tube is used to drain the contents of the stomach. It may be used for feeding a person who is unable to react normally.

16

Chapter

Radiopharmaceuticals

Introduction

A radiopharmaceutical is a chemical containing a radioactive isotope for use in humans for the purpose of diagnosis, mitigation or treatment of disease. Nuclear medicine is that branch of medicine which uses radioactive materials (radioisotopes and radiopharmaceuticals) to diagnose and treat diseases. Images obtained with a gamma camera represent the quantitative distribution of a radiopharmaceutical in the body. These examinations are particularly suited to examine the functions of the major organ systems in the body, as well as detect sites of inflammation/infection and tumor growth. Nuclear medicine procedures are also valuable aids to high resolution radiological techniques (i.e., CT and MRI) as they provide unique physiologic information about the patient while using small amounts of radioactivity with yield low total body radiation burdens.

The most common type of radioactive material used in nuclear medicine are gamma ray (γ) emitters such as technetium ^{m}–99, indium-111, thallium-201, gallium-67, iodine-123, etc. These radionuclides can be easily detected, quantified, and localized within the body with modern instrumentation. Scintillation gamma camera systems have attached dedicated computers which convert collected radioactive counts to functional images that allow visualization of functioning organs that are not routinely seen on X ray exams. Radionuclides (radiopharmaceuticals) can be administered orally, intravenously, or through intracavitary routes and they usually deliver lower doses of ionizing radiation than alternative radiographic techniques.

Both diagnostic examinations and radiotherapeutic treatments may be performed using radioactive materials. Many radionuclides emit negatively charged beta particles (electrons) with and without g rays (i.e., I-131, Sr-89, Re-186, P-32) and are used in nuclear medicine as therapeutic agents. Beta emitters when localized to a particular site such as the thyroid or a malignant tumor, can deposit energy and kill the offending tissue. Site specific therapy with beta emitters is presently an area of great interest in nuclear medicine.

Radioactive Half-Life

The radioactive half-life for a given radioisotope is the time for half the radioactive nuclei in any sample to undergo radioactive decay. After two half-lives, there will be one fourth the original sample, after three half-lives one eight the original sample, and so forth.

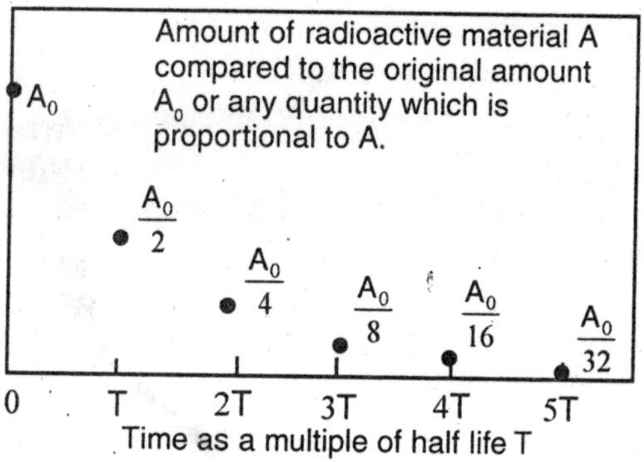

Units of Radioactivity

The number of decays per second, or activity, from a sample of radioactive nuclei is measured in becquerel (Bq), after Henri Becquerel. One decay per second equals one becquerel.

An older unit is the curie, named after Pierre and Marie Curie. One curie is approximately the activity of 1 gram of radium and equals (exactly) 3.7×10^{10} becquerel. The activity depends only on the number of decays per second, not on the type of decay, the energy of the decay products, or the biological effects of the radiation

Production of Radiopharmaceuticals

The production of Radiopharmaceuticals is expensive. It is based on four different methods :

- Nuclear fission(reactor breeding)
- Neutron activation process
- Charged particle induced reactions
- Radionuclide generator(chemical method)

Each method provides useful isotopes with differing characteristics for nuclear imaging.

Nuclear fission (reactor breeding) : In nuclear fission, the nuclei of atoms are split, causing energy to be released. The atomic bomb and nuclear reactors work by fission. The element uranium is the main fuel to undergo nuclear fission to produce energy since it has many favorable properties. Uranium nuclei is split, multiple neutrons are release which are used to split other uranium nuclei. This phenomenon is known as chain reaction.

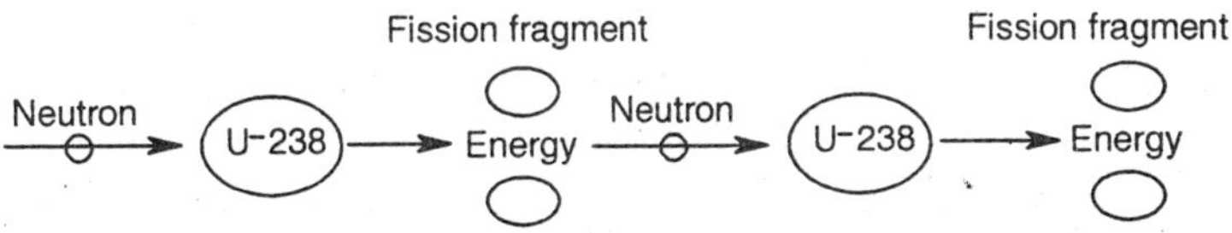

Nuclear fission takes place in the reactor core and induced by the slow neutron induced fission(break-up) of ^{235}U into medium mass nuclei. The most common radioisotopes produced by fission (with subsequent isotope separation base on different physical properties and chemical methods) are ^{99}Mo(which decays to $^{99}Tc^{m}$), ^{131}I and ^{133}Xe.

$$^{235}U + {^1n}_{thermal} \longrightarrow {^{236}U} \longrightarrow {^{99}Mo} + {^{134}Sn} + 3\,{^1n}$$

Neutron activation : It is based on capture reactions of thermal neutrons (produced in the reactor as consequence of the fission process) on stable isotopes which are positioned near the reaction core. Examples for radioisotopes via neutron capture are:

$$^{98}Mo + n \longrightarrow {^{99}Mo} + \gamma$$

$$^{50}Cr + n \longrightarrow {^{51}Cr} + \gamma$$

$$^{31}P + n \longrightarrow {^{32}P} + \gamma$$

$$^{32}S + n \longrightarrow {^{32}P} + p$$

The yield N_r, for the radioisotopes production over the time period t depends on the cross section σ [cm^2] of the neutron capture process, the neutron-flux ϕ [$cm^{-2}s^{-1}$], the number of target nuclei n_t and the decay constant $\lambda = \ln 2/T_{1/2}$.

$$N_r = \frac{\eta t.\phi.\alpha}{\lambda}.(1 - e^{-\lambda 4})$$

Disadvantage of this process is that the produced radioisotope is typically an isotope of target element, therefore chemical separation is not possible. This means that the (n, γi) produced radionucleate are not carrier free.

Charged particle induced reactions : It is based on the use of accelerators. Charged particles like protons, deutrons or alphas are accelerated in the energies between 1 to 100 MeV and bombarded a target material.

The most commonly used accelerator is cyclotron where the charged particles are accelerated by oscillating potentials perpendicular to deflecting magnetic field. The advantage of this method is the large difference in Z between the target material and the radionuclide. This allows good physical and chemical separation methods. ^{22}Sodium is prepared in this way by interaction of high velocity deuterons with magnesium.

$$24Mg\ (d, \sigma) \longrightarrow {}^{22}Na.$$

Radionuclide generators : It allows to separate chemically short lived radioactive daughter nuclei with good characteristics for medical imaging from long-lived radioactive parent nuclei. Typical techniques used are chromatographic absorption, distillation or phase separation. This method is in particular applied for the separation of rather short lived $^{99}Tc^m(T_{1/2} = 6hr)$ from the long lived $^{99}Mo(T_{1/2} = 27days)$.

Features of Radiochemical laboratory

A laboratory or facility used for investigation and handling of radioactive chemicals that provides a safe environment for the worker and the public. Features vary depending on the type of radioactive emissions to be handled, the quantity, the half-life, and the physical form (solid, liquid, gas, or powder). Special measures to minimize spread of contaminated material and to dispose of radioactive waste are required. Working surfaces should be smooth and easily washable to permit effective decontamination if necessary. Good ventilation and detectors for monitoring radiation and contamination on surfaces or people are also typical features.

Investigations utilizing only very small amounts (a few microcuries) of beta or gamma emitters which are not readily dispersed (no powders or volatile liquids) may sometimes be performed without special facilities on the bench top. In this case, precautions such as working on plastic-backed absorbent paper and wearing protective gloves and lab coat may be sufficient. A special bag or can for disposing of the paper and gloves as radioactive waste is required. If the radioactive isotopes are solely alpha-particle emitters, containment and isolation from direct contact are more serious concerns. Due to the limited penetration but high biological toxicity of alpha particles, it is essential to avoid ingestion or inhalation. For very small quantities, work may take place with double rubber gloves in a fume hood with appropriate filter. Generally, an enclosed glove box is used, situated inside a hood and maintained at negative pressure with respect to the face of the hood and the room. Sensors to monitor proper differential pressure and adequate airflow are usually used to assure containment and to generate an alarm if conditions degrade.

For work with pure beta-emitting isotopes, long-handled tongs or other tools are used for higher levels of radioactivity in order to shield the hands. Generally, since most beta emission is also accompanied by penetrating gamma emission, the entire work area must be enclosed in heavily shielded enclosures.

Hot laboratories contain walled enclosures for remotely handling larger quantities of gamma-emitting isotopes. A small enclosure is usually referred to as a cave, while large ones are called hot cells. Hot cells are usually equipped with remote manipulators and thick windows made from high-density lead glass.

Applications of Radionucleides

Radioisotopes are used in medicines in two different ways : (*i*) Radiation source in therapy. (*ii*) Radioactive tracers for diagnostic purposes.

Apart from this, they are also used in radiation sterilization. Thermolabile drugs like penicillin may be sterilized by radiation obtained from radionucleides. All microbes including spores are killed within seconds if targeted by radiation. Gamma rays from radioisotopes are used for this purpose. In therapeutic use of radioisotopes, the radiations emitted produce destructive effects on existing cells and prevent the formation of new cells and tissues. For this reason, radioisotope therapy is applied to those diseases in which extensive cellular metabolic malfunction exists, like cancer.

Use of radioisotopes, as therapeutic agents, depends mainly on their ability to ionize atoms. The energy measurement involved in radiations and resulting in ionization is expressed in millions of electron volts, called MeV. The strength or the energy of alpha, beta, and gamma rays is expressed as MeV. The radiation of short wavelength (gamma rays) has high penetrating power than long wavelength radiations (beta rays). Besides this, greater the MeV of the rays, more destructive it becomes to the surrounding tissues.

The diagnostic application include scintigraphy of organs, both static and dynamic imaging and as radioactive tracers. The static imaging gives the size and morphology of organ whereas dynamic imaging can be used for studying the functioning of organs.

Tracers acts as a spy left in the bulk material, which helps in detecting the path of the substance, mechanism of the reaction and processes. Some important radioisotopes used in medicine are:

Calcium (44Ca and 45Ca) : It is used to study bone structure and in the treatment of carcinoma of bones.

Carbon (14C) : It is most widely used in various studies to detect reaction mechanism, metabolism of carbohydrate and fats, drug excretion, decomposition of pharmaceutical products.

Cobalt (60Co) : This agent emits beta and gamma rays and is used in therapy where X-rays are used. It is also used for the sterilization of surgical materials and gamma rays are used to sterilize the dressings.

Cyanocobalamine (57Co) : It is a cyanocobalamine containing 57Co. It is used in the diagnosis of pernicious anemia.

Gold (198Au) solution : It is a cherry red, colloidal solution of radioactive gold (198Au), which is sterilized by autoclaving. It emits beta particles and gamma rays. It is used as a neoplastic suppressant. It is also used in estimation of reticulo-endothelial activity.

Hydrogen (2H, 3H) : Deuterium and tritium are useful to determine total body water.

Iron (55Fe, 59Fe) : Iron is used in the research studies related to the utilization and absorption of iron salts. It is also used to measure the cell life span of R.B.C.

Nitrogen (13N, 15N) : It is useful in investigations of amino acids and protein metabolism and also in the studies of nitrogen fixation by plants.

Oxygen (17O, 18O) : These are useful in studies of organic reactions and photosynthesis etc.

Sodium (22Na, 24Na) : It is used for estimation of extracellular fluid, blood circulation rate, and studies related to thc cell permeability, excretion and distribution of water etc.

Chromium (51Cr) : It is a radioactive chromium ion in the form of Na2Cr51O4. It is used to study red cell volume and its survival time.

Sodium iodide (131I) : It is used in the form of capsule and solution. It emits beta and gamma rays. It is mainly used as a diagnostic and therapeutic agent in thyroid conditions and myxodema.

Sodium phosphate (32P) solution : It is used in the form of sodium acid phosphate in the treatment of polycythemia vera to decrease the rate of formation of the erythrocytes. It is also used in the treatment of chronic granulocytic leukemia.

Biological effects of radiation

Ionization and excitation of molecules in the body cause abnormal chemical reactions. The effect of abnormal chemical reactions depend on number of factors such as:

(*i*) Penetration power of radiation.

(*ii*) Energy of radiation

(*iii*) Particular tissue and the surface area exposed.

Actively dividing cells are the most sensitive if exposed to radiations as is the case in cells ofreproductive organs, blood forming tissues, skin and hair roots.

(*iv*) Dose of radiation, and

(*v*) Time of the exposure.

The destructive effects of radiation include inactivation of essential enzymes, coagulation of protein, destruction of nucleic acid and production of histamine like substances. Damage to only a small fraction of the molecules in a living cell is sufficient to produce serious effects.

Some of the damage caused by radiation is due to an indirect effect. Action on water molecules leads to the production of free radicals.

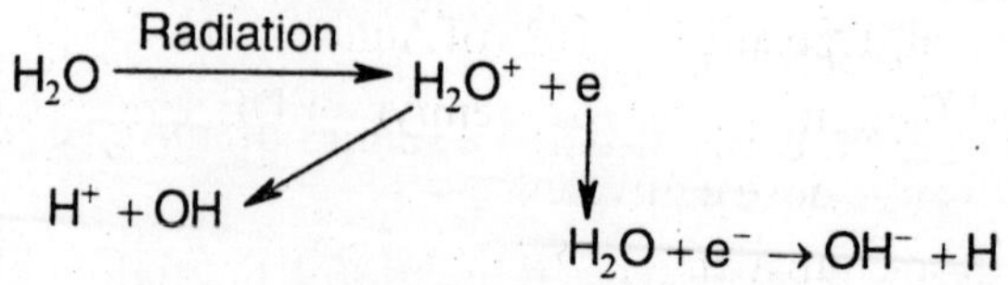

The free radical .OH and H. may react

$$^{\bullet}OH + {^{\bullet}OH} \rightarrow 2O_2$$

$$H^{\bullet} + H^{\bullet} \rightarrow H_2$$

If atmospheric oxygen is present, then

$$H^{\bullet} + O_2 \rightarrow H^{\bullet}O_2$$

$$2H^{\bullet}O_2 \rightarrow H_2O_2 + O_2$$

The powerful oxidizing activity of the hydrogen peroxide, $^{\bullet}OH$, and $H^{\bullet}O_2$ free radical is responsible for some of the destructive effects of radiation.

Skin damages : A short exposure to the intense radiation produces erythema. Longer exposure can cause brittleness and dryness (due to destruction of sebaceous gland, loss of hair (due to damage to the hair follicles) and if the dose is very large, then burns may take place. The latter heal very slowly and occasionally become malignant.

Somatic effects : Some effects like cataract, severe anemia, leukemia and cancer are visible after two months upto many years after exposure to radiation. Cancer tends to occur in tissues severally damaged by radiation. The latent period is very long and often exceeds twenty years.

Genetic effects : Radiation has two effects on reproductive cells. It can damage the chromosomes and increase the chance of gene manipulation. The former effect is not very important as it is caused by long exposure to low intensity X- and gamma rays. The mutation will be inherited by future generation and most are believed to be harmful.

Maximum permissible radiation dose limits

ADULT OCCUPATIONAL EXPOSURE

Whole body	5 rem/yr TEDE 0.05 Sv/yr
Skin of whole body or extremity	50 rem/yr TEDE 0.5 Sv/yr
Eye	15 rem/yr LDE 0.15 Sv/yr
Embryo/fetus	0.5 rem/gestation period TEDE 0.005 Sv

Minors occupational exposure	10% of Adult limits
Member of general public	0.1 rem/yr TEDE 1 m Sv/yr

TEDE = Total effective dose equivalent

SDE = Shallow dose equivalent

LDE = Lens of eye dose equivalent

Ssieverts (Sv) is dose unit for biological tissue, where 1 Sv is equal to 1 joule per kilogram.

ALARA PHILOSOPHY

Current scientific evidence concedes that there may not be a risk-free level of radiation exposure. Therefore, in addition to providing an upper limit on a person's permissible radiation exposure, it also requires that its licensees maintain occupational exposures as low as reasonably achievable (ALARA). This means that every activity involving exposure to radiation should be planned so as to minimize unnecessary exposure to individual workers and the worker population. All experimental procedures should be reviewed with the objective of reducing unnecessary exposures.

Protection Against Radiation

A. External radiation protection principles

Time : Radiation doses are directly proportional to the exposure time in the field. If the time spent in a given radiation field is doubled, the worker's dose is doubled. Therefore, to limit radiation doses, the time spent in the field must be limited.

$$\text{Radiation Dose} \times (\text{Time in field})$$

Distance : By far the best shielding against radioactivity is GAUSS' LAW: the radiation dose received from a source is inversely proportional to the square of the distance of separation. If the distance is increased ten-fold the exposure will be cut down to one percent. Thus, the distance of separation between a person and a "point" source has a relatively greater influence on dose than the time factor.

$$\text{Radiation dose} \times 1/(\text{Distance of Separation})^2$$

All localized sources are labelled with their activity *at a given distance*, for instance "10 *mr/h* at 1 *m*." If one keeps at least 10 *m* away from such a source, one will receive less than 0.1 *mR* per hr, which is not worrisome.

Shielding : Any substance may serve to attenuate radiation to acceptable levels provided sufficient thickness is used. Certain materials, however, are more effective in shielding certain types of radiation.

Alpha particles are stopped by an ordinary sheet of paper or a few inches of air.

Beta particles although more penetrating than alpha, can be absorbed readily and completely. Figure 4 shows the shielding required for complete absorption of beta rays of various energies in various substances. For example, beta rays of one million electron volts (MeV) are completely absorbed by 0.15 cm of aluminum.

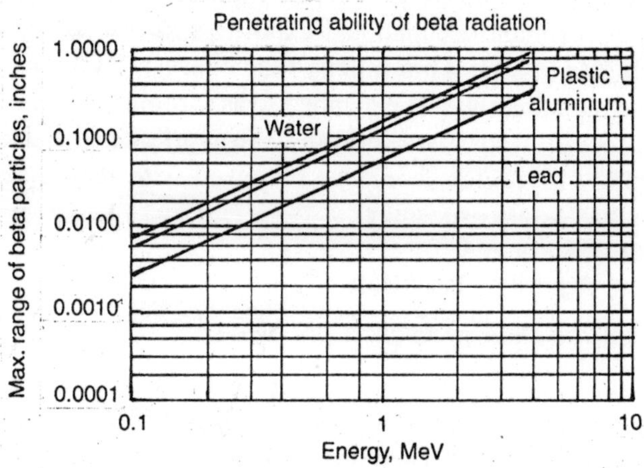

Gamma rays and x-rays of a single energy (monoenergetic) are attenuated exponentially; therefore, theoretically it is not possible to attenuate the radiation completely, although the exposure rate can be reduced by any desired factor. Thus, if a certain thickness of absorber, the half-value layer (HVL), reduces the dose to one-half the initial amount, then a thickness of three such layers will reduce the dose to one-eighth (½ × ½ × ½) the initial amount. Similarly three tenth-value layers (TVL) will reduce the dose to 1/1000 of the initial amount (1/10 × 1/10 × 1/10). Shielding materials of high density and high atomic number, such as lead, are generally the most effective absorbers or shields for x- and gamma rays. Thus, less thickness and weight per square foot is required for such materials. However, steel, concrete, brick, or other materials can provide the same degree of protection if used in appropriately greater thicknesses.

B. Internal radiation protection principles

An internal radiation hazard exists when radionuclides can enter the body by ingestion or inhalation, through wounds, or by direct absorption through intact skin. The radiation doses are often difficult to cvaluate and depend on many factors such as the physical and chemical form of the material, the mode of entry, and the individual's metabolism. A certain quantity of radioactive material within the body represents a greater hazard than the same activity as an external source because the tissue is irradiated continuously until the material has decayed or been eliminated. Even weakly penetrating radiations such as low-encrgy beta particles present a hazard since all their energy will be dissipated in the tissue. The principal means of protection from internal radiation is containment of the radioactive source. Control measures must be taken to prevent the contamination of working surfaces, equipment, and personnel. The following covers some of these safety precautions and procedures.

C. General precautions and safety procedures when working with radioactive materials

1. Be familiar with the particular clinical or experimental procedure being performed. Never perform extensive radiochemical work with hazardous levels of material until the procedure has been tested by a "dry run" to preclude unexpected complications.
2. Keep radioactive and non-radioactive work separate as much as possible by maintaining designated and labeled areas on the bench top and in the laboratory.
3. Cover work surfaces with absorbent padding that has a plastic backing to protect furniture and facilitate clean up. Use stainless steel or plastic trays to help control liquids if these are spilled.
4. When working with radioactive materials, wear a laboratory coat and plastic or rubber gloves for protection of clothes and skin. To avoid the spread of contamination, remove gloves at the work area. Change gloves frequently to prevent the spread of contamination. Do not handle faucets, light switches, door knobs, telephones, etc., with contaminated gloves. Special protection may be required for open cuts or wounds.
5. Monitor yourself for contamination at frequent intervals when working with radioactive materials. Monitoring should include hands, body, shoes, and protective clothing.

6. Clean up after yourself. Do not leave the laboratory contaminated or in a mess. Check all work areas for contamination. Before leaving the laboratory, wash your hands thoroughly.
7. Never pipette radioactive solutions by mouth. Mechanical devices must be used. Push-button pipetters with disposable tips are strongly recommended.
8. To prevent accidental ingestion of radioactive materials, do not eat, drink, smoke, store or prepare food, or apply cosmetics in restricted areas.
9. Do not handle sources of high radioactivity directly with your fingers. Use tongs.
10. Observe time, distance, shielding, and contamination control while working with radioactive materials or while in a radiation area.
11. If you are designated to wear a personnel (TLD) monitoring badge, you should wear it at all times when working with or near radioactive materials for which the badge is appropriate.
12. Have containers for radioactive waste and contaminated glassware at the work location. Avoid transporting contaminated articles from the work area through clean laboratory areas. Shield the waste containers as required to prevent unnecessary exposure.
13. Confine work with gaseous, volatile, or dust-forming radioactive material to fume hoods or glove boxes, if appropriate.
14. Label containers of radioactive material clearly, indicating radionuclide, activity, compound, date, and radiation level, if applicable.

Radioisotope thermoelectric generator

A radioisotope thermoelectric generator (RTG) is an electrical generator which obtains its power from radioactive decay. In such a device, the heat released by the decay of a suitable radioactive material is converted into electricity by the Seebeck effect using an array of thermocouples. RTGs can be considered as a type of battery and have been used as power sources in satellites, space probes and unmanned remote facilities. RTGs are usually the most desirable power source for unmanned or unmaintained situations needing a few hundred watts or less of power for durations too long for fuel cells, batteries and generators to provide economically, and in places where solar cells are not viable.

The radioactive material used in RTGs must have several characteristics:

- The half-life must be long enough that it will produce energy at a relatively continuous rate for a reasonable amount of time. However, at the same time, the half-life needs to be short enough so that it decays sufficiently quickly to generate a usable amount of heat. Typical half-lives for radioisotopes used in RTGs are therefore several decades, although isotopes with shorter half-lives could be used for specialized applications.
- For spaceflight use, the fuel must produce a large amount of energy per mass and volume (density). Density and weight are not as important for terrestrial use, unless there are size restrictions.
- It should produce high energy radiation that has low penetration, preferably alpha radiation. Beta radiation can give off considerable amounts of Gamma/X-ray radiation through bremsstrahlung secondary radiation production, thus requiring heavy shielding. Isotopes must not produce significant amounts of gamma, neutron radiation or penetrating radiation in general through other decay modes or decay chain products.

The first two criteria limit the number of possible fuels to fewer than 30 atomic isotopes within the entire table of nuclides. Plutonium-238, curium-244 and strontium-90 are the most often cited candidate isotopes, but other isotopes such as polonium-210, promethium-147, caesium-137, cerium-144, ruthenium-106, cobalt-60, curium-242 and thulium isotopes have also been studied.

Section-II

Clinical Pharmacy

17
Chapter

Clinical Pharmacy

Pharmacy contribution in recent years has increased considerably beyond drug manufacture and distribution in advance countries. It is only due to greater involvement of a pharmacist in drug related decision and patient care activities. Physician diagnoses the disease and suggests the drug therapy. The pharmacist performs both non-clinical and clinical functions. Non-clinical functions involve the manufacturing and distribution of drugs. In the clinical function, pharmacist is often called a clinical pharmacist, advises the physician about the dosage regimen and possible drug interaction. He also counsels the patient about the disease, adverse drug reactions and other clinical concern.

Clinical pharmacy is a branch which involves the participation of clinical pharmacist in drug therapy decisions in patient care areas.

Objectives of Clinical Pharmacy

The objective of this discipline is to promote the safe and effective use of drugs in patients in collaboration with other professionals responsible for health care and, more specifically, the provision of drug information to other health professionals; the acquisition of medication histories and the use of the pharmacotherapeutic profile of patients; monitoring of treatments; the provision of information and advice about medication to the patient; participation in emergency medical care; participation in reviewing the use of drugs; the provision of internal educational programs for physicians, nurses and other healthcare professionals.

Functions of clinical Pharmacy

Major functions of clinical pharmacy are as follows :

1. Preparation of patient medication history chart : Patient prescription and non-prescription drugs, allergic disorder and adverse drug reactions including patient compliance are recorded in the medication history chart. It helps the physician in making decision on current treatment in the patient best interest.
2. Monitoring the patient's response to the current medication is done in order to maximize benefits and to either medication problems arising or to help their early recognition and correction if they do arise.
3. It involves in increasing the knowledge about the disease and their drug therapy. He can guide the patient for proper use of drug therapy and possible drug interaction. He can also advice for the drug compliance.
4. Participation in medical emergencies.
5. It also provides the provision of consultation in various areas like total parenteral nutrition, intravenous therapy, clinical pharmacokinetics, selection of drug therapy and determination of therapeutic end point.
6. Management of chronic diseases.
7. Clinical pharmacist participates in clinical drug inestigation along with other medical staff members.
8. Clinical pharmacist is involved in drug administration and drug distribution in the patient care area.
9. Clinical pharmacist is involved in the education of medical, pharmacy and nursing personnel in the patient care areas.
10. Clinical pharmacist involves in detection and reporting of adverse drug reaction and drug interaction.
11. Clinical pharmacist involves in conduction of drug use reviews and participation in patient care audits.
12. Clinical pharmacist has the responsibility to communicate the development made in drug delivery system and clinical pharmacy services.

Status of Clinical Pharmacy in India

Due to introduction of pharmacy practice education decade before in India, there has been a paradigm shift in the practice of pharmacy in the country. In spite of this, pharmacy practice education faces many challenges before it can transform the pharmaceutical care practice in India from a product-oriented approach to patient-oriented care.

Pharmacy education in India is mainly industry oriented. The curriculum at the undergraduate level is more or less designed for preparing students towards industry rather than for patient-oriented services like hospital, clinical and community pharmacy. To train the graduate pharmacists to provide patient-oriented services, a pharmacy practice course was started at a postgraduate level. Pharmacy practice curriculum enters its tenth year in India since its beginning in 1997. The curriculum trains the postgraduates in rational therapeutics, patient counselling, pharmacovigilance, therapeutic drug monitoring, clinical research and toxicology to name a few. With the efforts being on introducing the advanced clinical-based courses of the doctor of pharmacy (PharmD) degree in India, there is a need to contemplate where the profession stands at this juncture. As of today pharmacy practice is at a crossroads in India, facing numerous challenges that need to be addressed before marching further. This letter is an effort to identify deficiencies, vis-a-vis regulatory requirement and evaluate the current status of pharmacy practice education in India.

The decade long journey of pharmacy practice curriculum in India provides some key insights :

1. **The profession is restricted only to the hospitals linked to a pharmacy practice school.** With the completion of a decade there are few pharmacy schools providing specialization in pharmacy practice. Due to lack of job avenues, prospective postgraduates cannot opt to work as a clinical pharmacist in Indian hospitals as the value of clinical pharmacy services is not recognized.
2. **Regulatory framework does not recognize the need for clinical pharmacist at the national level.** There are no regulatory guidelines for having qualified clinical pharmacists in an Indian hospital. Even if the regulations are framed in due course, a point to ponder is whether there will be any experienced pharmacists left to practice the clinical set up as there is a mass migration of trained clinical pharmacist to pharmaceutical industry. Though clinical pharmacists have gained the confidence and acceptance of the medical fraternity, that acceptance alone will not help to overcome the shortcomings, like lack of a regulatory framework of scarce job opportunities as a clinical pharmacist. Pharmacy councils and professional leaders need to take initiative by lobbying with relevant government authorities to create a position in the hospital set-up where a trained clinical pharmacist can fit in.

3. **Exodus of trained clinical pharmacists toward industry as there is almost no opportunity in the hospital setting.** As there is no recognition of the job done by the clinical pharmacist at the regulatory level, the profession failed in to create job opportunities in hospitals for qualified clinical pharmacy postgraduates. Students are forced to either seek jobs in industries (clinical research) or continue in academies, at times teaching subjects which are out of scope of clinical pharmacy (as not many university hospitals have pharmacy practice school). The last option being to move to countries like USA, UK, Australia where the pharmacy profession is well recognized.
4. **The need for adding industry relevant topics in course curriculum – Dilemma of dilution vs. evolution.** There is a widening gap between the number of students graduating from pharmacy practice institutions and the number actually employed as pharmacy practitioners. There is a need to take key steps to either create a niche for clinical pharmacy professionals in the hospital or make them competent to take up other challenging jobs in the industry. There is a need for introducing specific roles that include training in pharmacogenomics, pharmacokinetic-pharmacodynamics and medical informatics, which are job-oriented skills. Before the academic move to the next step of bringing PharmD courses, there is a need to augment the acceptability for existing courses. In an evidence-based health service, it is not just sufficient to propose new roles for clinical pharmacist without adequate evidence of benefits. Services should not only be clinically cost effective but also acceptable to patients and other health care colleagues.

This situation helps the profession to learn the difficulties in implementing patient-oriented services when the health care system does not recognise the need for clinically trained pharmacists. The experience in the past decade helped to understand the lacunae within the profession, especially on the regulatory side. This situation calls for the sustained effort by academic leaders to work with government authorities to bring suitable changes in regulation that will help the profession grow towards patient care. Working on regulatory issues with the respective government authorities is an important task for profession leaders as the regulatory environment is one of the important factors that determine the growth of health professionals like pharmacy.

To summarize, clinical pharmacy education in India after a decade is at a crossroad. The pharmacy educators are in a dilemma as to whether the course will evolve by incorporating industry relevant components or progress into a clinically relevant course with the help of regulatory changes. This dilemma may resolve with time.

18
Chapter

Modern Dispensing Aspects

The significant advances in development of new therapeutic agent have made the most of disease curable provided the patient takes the drugs in a prescribed manner. It means that patient should understand well how to take the medications. If he don't take the medication according to the direction provided deliberately or innocently, the treatment becomes useless. To describe this fact, the term '*patient non-compliance*' is coined.

Patient Compliance

When the patient does not follow the instruction given by a doctor or mentioned on label for the usage of medication to cure or control the disease, the patient can be said as non-compliant. Some researchers use the term 'adherence' instead of compliance.

The term non-compliance or non-adherance not only include the drug therapy but also the failure to obey instruction on other aspects of health care such as dieting, exercise and smoking or drinking habits.

It is difficult to assess the acceptable level of compliance or non-compliance. Ideally it would be assessed on a biological basis such as the point below which desired therapeutic or prophylactic result is unlikely to be achieved. It may be possible to define the term compliance arbitrarily as follows :

$$\% \text{ compliance} = \frac{\text{NDP} - \text{NME}}{\text{NDP}} \times 100$$

NDP is the number of doses prescribed.

NME is the number of medication.

Any valve less than 90% indicate the non-compliance.

The situations most commonly associated with non-compliance with drug therapy include failure to have the prescription filled, lapses in the doses, errors of dosage, errors in the time of administration of drug, premature discontinuation of the drug, and taking a drug for the wrong purpose. It is tried to correlate the non-compliance with different variables like age, sex, education, severity of disease and others. It has been shown that one-third of the patients failed to comply with instructions in short term treatment but in long term treatment (chronic illness), the rate of non-compliance is approximately 50%. It is concluded that 25-60% elderly patients are non-compliant to the directions provided by the doctors. It is judged that one-third of patients on chlorpropamide take less than half of the prescribed therapy.

Reasons for Non-Compliance

Various reasons for non-compliance are as follows :

(i) **Inappropriate packaging :** Sometimes design or fize of container makes the medicament in accessible for, e.g. the presence of arthritis or the loss of fine finger movement in parkinsonism will make the medicines inaccessible if the size of the container is too small or the cap is difficult to remove. Many elderly patients have difficulty with the unit dose packs or foil wrappings while taking out the medicament.

(ii) **Poor labelling :** Poorly handwritten labels are a major source of medication error as it is difficult to read/follow for the patient. Many prescription items bears directions which are inadequate like 'take when required', one as 'formerly or as directed'. Such advice is meaningless and serious discrepancies may exist between the doctor's intention and the patient interpretation.

(iii) **Social isolation :** It is beneficial to ensure that the medication is taken as directed. If the patient is socially isolated as in schizophrenia, then there is more chance of non-compliance. This is the reason that such patient are admitted in the hospital for treatment.

(iv) **Complex therapeutic regimes :** There is more chance of non-compliance if the patient receive more than three different preparations at a time. Such patient frequently suffer from illness for which multiple drug therapy is compulsory due to non-compliance reason. In multiple drug therapy, there may be an error in time of administration of drug.

(v) **Mental illness :** Sometime patient are mentally confused and may forget to take an occasional dose of medicament or a loss of memory a few minutes after drug intake may result in unnecessary duplication of dosage. Many patients mix a variety of tablets in a single bottle and they feel in need of dose, the first tablet to fall out of the bottle is taken.

(vi) **Nature of medication :** Complication of old age, when eyesight and manual dexterity may be falling, make the drug preparation an important factor in terms of compliance. Extremely small tablets may cause problem as they are difficult to identify or handle while large size tablets are frequently difficult to swallow.

Unpleasant taste, odour or colour also cause non-compliance particularly among the children.

(vii) **Side effects :** Side effects of drug may cause non-compliance. For example, tricyclic antidepressants make the patient feelings worse before any beneficial effect is realized.

(viii) **Lack of doctor/patient report :** The attitude of the doctor strongly affects the patient compliance. It is observed that when the patient is satisfied with the medical consultation, he follows the direction to maximum extent. By chance, if he is dissatisfied, he becomes casual to follow the instructions.

(ix) **Inadequate patient education :** Lack of proper advice or lack of patient education is a prime reason for non-compliance.

The patient may use tablets as suppositories or suppositories as tablets, use antibiotic capsules in the ear or swallow the ampoule of medicament.

Importance of Non-Compliance

The drug response is affected by various factors including compliance of patient. The consequences of patient non-compliance with the treatment depend largely on specific medication and the underlying clinical status of the patients :

(i) There will be lack of therapeutic response if drug is not administered timely. It may initiate the unnecessary prescription for higher dosage or ultimately a re-assessment of the diagnosis.

Higher dosage may cause harmful effect due to excess pharmacological effect. Re-assessment of diagnosis leads to delaying of treatment.

(ii) If the patient does not complete the short term course of antibiotics, generally course, especially in tuberculosis therapy, lapses in the dose result in development of resistance. Tuberculosis patient may develop resistance if there is lapses in the dose. It occurs when patient is not compliant with the treatment.

(iii) Non-compliance with anticonvulsant drugs therapy results in uncontrolled seizures which may cause death.

(iv) Omission of a few doses of insulin or clonidine may be life threatening. Lapses in clonidine dose, cause rebound hypertension which may cause angina.

(v) Failure to take even a single dose of the contraceptive pill can result in unwanted pregnancy.

(vi) Digoxin, hydrochlorothiazide and potassium chloride are prescribed together to the cardiac patient. Potassium chloride is used to compensate the loss of potassium occur with diuretic therapy. If the patient is non-compliant to potassium chloride, he becomes more sensitive to action of digoxin.

(vii) Overdosage of medicament may cause serious health hazards. Sometimes, the patient takes two or three doses simultaneously by assuming that he will get better relief or get relief more quickly which may result in severe toxic effects.

(viii) Some non-compliance may result from improper administration or using a medication for the wrong purpose. This problem is common in rectal, vaginal or ophthalmic dosage form. Many patients use the drug in a similar manner, as adopted by friends and relatives. This type of practice may be dangerous for health.

Role of Pharmacist in Improving Compliance

Generally both the physician and the pharmacist have the opportunity to interest directly with the patient and give proper explanation about the drug therapy. The effective communication will encourage the compliance. The pharmacist has a particularly better opportunity to encourage compliance since his advice accompanies the actual dispensing of the medication and he is usually the last health professional to see the patient prior to the time the medication is to be used. In addition, the patient may find it easier to establish rapport with the pharmacist and this is reflected by many occasions in which a patient asks a pharmacist about his disease or medication because of reluctance to discuss these matters with the physician. Patient compliance with drug therapy is mainly dependent upon the effective communication of instruction, necessary for correct use of medication or counselling. It is part of the clinical pharmacy practice to give maximum benefits to the patient. It includes the direction given by the pharmacist to the patient regarding the prescribed drugs.

Routine counselling of all patients is both undesirable and impractical. Priority should be given to the patient where :

(i) prophylactic treatment is required in the absence of symptoms (e.g. tuberculosis).

(ii) the drugs in use have a low margin of safety (e.g. warfarin).

(iii) premature withdrawal from treatment causes serious consequences (e.g. corticocoids), and

(iv) long term therapy is indicated for a chronic disease (e.g. epilepsy).

Pharmacist should conveyed the information in a manner which the patient can easily understand. Common language and general terms should be used in a manner which is reassuring rather than threatening.

The basic information which are given by the pharmacist during counselling include :

(i) the purpose of medication,

(ii) method of administration,

(iii) time of drug intake,

(iv) common side effects which may be classified as (a) those which will disappear, (b) those which must be tolerated, advice may be given on management, (c) those which warrant the attention of doctors or pharmacists,

(v) storage advice,

(vi) specific activities to avoid,

(vii) about interaction with food, alcohol or smoking, and

(viii) adverse drug reactions, e.g. allergy which may occur with the use of some drugs like penicillins and sulphonamides.

Another important aspects of patient counselling is to emphasize the changes in drug therapy which have occurred during the patient stay in hospital. In addition, measures should be taken to discourage the drug hoarding.

Medication History

An accurate and complete patient medication history is beneficial to the physician in making decisions on current treatment and is thus in the patient's best interest. The medication history alerts to previous adverse effects, potential adverse reactions or allergies, or possible interactions affecting the validity of laboratory tests. The medication history also informs about patient's self prescribing habits and patient compliance toward the treatment.

Pharmacists are capable of obtaining detailed medication histories due to his better knowledge. In order to obtain the necessary information in comprehensive form, the pharmacist should conduct the interview in predetermined systematic and flexible way; first of all, the pharmacist should acquaint himself with the patient charts so that he is familiar with the present medical status and background details of the patient. The pharmacist could start the interview by introducing himself and explaining the purpose of the interview. Get the name, address, age etc. of the patient and then collect the past history. Direct or indirect, questions can be asked around main subject areas such as prescribed medication, self medication, allergies, sensitivities or undesirable effect of the drug, compliance to prescribed medication, smoking, drinking and eating habits. The terminology used in the patient interview should be easily understandable by the patient, e.g. heart burn, indigestion and flatulence. Pharmacist can explain the difficult terms if not followed by the patient. Other areas to question include constipation, diarrhoea, cough and cold, hay fever, allergies, vitamins, tonics, eye, ear and skin preparations.

Towards the end of the interviews, when hopefully the pharmacist has the patient's confidence, question can be asked to ascertain the patient's medication compliance pattern. This may be a valuable information which could significantly help in the treatment of the patient.

All the informations, collected from interview, are then recorded in the patient medication interview form (its copy should be transferred to physician).

Instructions for Some Commonly Used Drugs

Non-compliance is resulted when direction given by the physician/ pharmacist is not clear, for example "take as directed" or "as required". The correct advice in a simple language helps in improving to a greater extent. Some common examples are illustrated here.

	Drugs	*Instructions*
1.	Salicylates	Do not take on empty stomach
2.	Tetracyclines	Do not take with milk or antacids
3.	Antacid tablets	Chew, do not swallow
4.	Bisascodyl (Dulcolax)	Do not take antacid or milk within one hour of drug administration
5.	MAO inhibitors	Avoid cheese, chocolate, alcoholic beverages and liver or yeast extract
6.	Antidiabetics	Avoid alcoholic beverages
7.	Diazepam	This drug may cause drowsiness so : (1) Do not work with dangerous machinery and do not drive a vehicle which may require you to be alert and (2) Do not drink alcoholic beverages
8.	Liquid paraffin (lubricant laxative)	Do not use for prolonged time
9.	Diphenhydramine	It may cause sedation, so don't drive vehicle
10.	Phenylbutazone and oxyphenbutazone	Do not take on empty stomach
11.	Vaginal contraceptive suppositories	Insert about 10 minutes before coitus, each suppository remains effective for 1 hr
12.	Spermicidal jellies and creams	Creams and jellies should be inserted 10 to 30 minutes before intercourse and must remain in vagina for 6-8 hours afterwards
13.	Ampicillin	Take this medicine in an empty stomach at least one hour before or 2 hours after food

19 Chapter

Commonly Used Terminology in the Practice of Medicine

Related with dosage form :

1. *Liquid dosage forms* : It includes (1) solution, (2) emulsion, (3) suspension.
2. *Solid dosage forms* : It includes (1) tablet, (2) capsules, (3) cachets etc.
3. *Semi-solid dosage forms* : It includes (1) ointments, (2) creams, (3) gels, (4) pastes.

On the basis of the route of administration, the dosage forms can be divided into :

1. *Dosage forms meant for parenteral administration* : It includes all injectables preparation and implants.
2. *Dosage forms meant for oral administration* : It includes (1) tablets, (2) capsules, (3) powders, (4) granules, (5) liquid mixtures, (6) suspension, (7) syrup, etc.
3. *Dosage forms meant for external administration* : It includes (1) ointments, (2) creams, (3) lotions, (4) liniments, (5) application, (6) paints, (7) dusting powder, (8) gels, (9) sprays, etc.
4. *Dosage forms meant for installation into eyes, ear and nose* : Ear drops, nasal drops, eye drops, ointment, etc.
5. *Dosage forms meant for body cavities* : (1) Nasal bogies, (2) suppositories, (3) pessaries, (4) rectal tablets, (5) vaginal tablets, (6) enemas, (7) douches.
6. *Dosage meant for inhalation* : (1) Aerosal and spray, (2) nasal inhalation, (3) oral inhalation, (4) insufflation, etc.

Aerosols	Aerosols are suspensions of liquid globules or fine solid particles in a gaseous vehicle.
Application	They are liquid or semi-liquid preparations applied to skin surface.
Aromatic waters	Automatic waters are aqueous saturated solution of volatile oil or other aromatic volatile substances, used as flavouring agent.
Cachets	Cachets are related to capsules as they provide an edible container for oral administration of nauseous and disagreeable powders or solid drugs.
Capsules	Capsules are solid unit dosage forms in which the drug or medicament is enclosed either in a hard or soft gelatin shell. Capsules can be made to give effect for a long duration (sustained released form).
Creams	Creams are non-greasy semisolid preparations. They are either o/w or w/o type, meant for external use.
Collodions	Collodions preparations are prepared in volatile solvents such as ether and alcohol meant for external use only.
Douches	Douches is an aqueous solution meant for introduction into one of the body cavities either for medicinal treatment or for hygienic purposes.
Draughts	Draughts are liquid oral preparations or liquid medicaments of dispensed/packed in a single dose container for one or sometimes two time use only.
Dusting powder	Dusting powders applied to various parts of the body as antiseptic, astringent, antiperspirants, antipurities, absorbents, protectives and lubricants.
Elixirs	These preparations are clear, pleasantly flavoured sweetened and attractively coloured hydro-alcoholic liquids intended for oral administration.
Emulsions	Emulsions are biphasic liquid or semi-solid dosage forms in which two immiscible liquids or substances such as an oil and water are miscible by the addition of an emulsifying agent.
Ear drops	Ear drops are sterile liquid preparations meant for instillation into the ears with the help of a dropper.

Eye drops	Eye drops are sterile isotonic liquid preparations or suspensions meant for instillation into the eyes.
Enemas	Enemas are liquids in the form of solution or suspension or o/w emulsion and are intended for rectal administration. They may contain medicament, lubricant, emollient, etc.
Extracts	Extracts are concentrated preparation of drugs (drug and menstrum ratio is 1 : 1).
Gargles	Gargles are aqueous liquid preparations used externally. They are used to prevent or treat throat infection.
Gels	Gels are semi-solid colloidal suspensions meant for external use.
Granules	They are the solid medicaments which have unpleasant taste.
Implants	Implants are small tablets meant for insertion under the skin by giving a small surgical cut into the skin.
Inhalations	Inhalations are liquid dosage forms of volatile substances, used to relieve congestion and inflammation of the respiratory tract.
Insufflations	These are finely divided powdered medicaments, which are introduced into body cavities, such as throat, ear, nost and tooth socket.
Irrigations	Irrigation preparations are used to treat infection of nose, urinary bladder and vagina.
Jellies	Jellies are non-greasy, transparent or translucent semi-solid preparations meant for external use only.
Liniments	Liniments are liquid or semi-liquid or semi-solid preparations applied on the skin.
Lotions	Lotions are liquid preparations in the form of solution or suspension intended for application to the skin without friction. They are also used as mouth wash and gargles.
Lozenges	These are solid dosage forms usually, sweetish in taste meant for mouth and throat for the slow release of medicaments.
Mixtures	There are medicated liquid preparations meant for oral administration.

Mouth washes	These are liquid preparations intended for oral hygiene to treat mouth infection.
Nasal drops	These are the sterile medicated liquid preparations meant for instillation into nose.
Ointments	Ointments are the semi-solid greasy preparations applied on the skin.
Paints	Paints are the viscous liquid preparations applied to the skin or mucous membrane of mouth and throat with the help of the cotton.
Pastes	Pastes are semi-solid preparations meant for external use only.
Pessaries	These are solid dosage forms for insertion into vagina to treat infections.
Pills	Pills are solid oral dosage forms of medicament. They are spherical or ovoid in shape.
Poultices	These are semi-solid paste like preparations meant for external use only.
Powders	Powders are solid dosage forms of medicament intended for oral administration or for external use.
Spirits	Spirits are alcoholic or hydro-alcoholic solutions of volatile oils or other aromatic compounds.
Sprays	Sprays are liquid preparations intended for spraying to the mucosal of nose or throat with the help of an atomiser or nebuliser.
Solutions	These are the liquid dosage forms in which medicament and other ingredients of the preparation are dissolved in the vehicle.
Suppositories	Suppositories are conical or avoid shaped solid dosage forms meant for insertion into rectum or other body cavities other than mouth.
Suspension	Suspensions are the biphasic liquid or semi solid dosage forms of medicament in which the finely divided solid particles are dispersed or suspended in a liquid or semi-solid vehicles.
Syrups	Syrups are the aqueous liquid preparations intended for oral administration in which the vehicle used is a concentrated aqueous solution of sucrose or other sugars (62 gm/100 ml).

Tablets	Tablets are the solid unit dosage forms of medicament administered by oral route.
Tinctures	These are alcoholic or hydro-alcoholic liquid preparations containing the active constituents of vegetable drugs (drug and mentrum ratio is 1 : 4).
Vehicles	These are the substances in which the medicament is either dissolved or suspended.

Related with Pharmacological Basis

Antibiotics	A substance, produced by or derived from a microorganism, that destroys or inhibits the growth of other microorganisms. Antibiotics are used to treat infections caused by organisms that are sxensitive to them, usually bacteria or fungi.
Amoebiasis	Intestinal or extra intestinal infection caused by protozoal organisms, *Entamoeba histolytica*.
Anthelmintics	Any drug or chemical agent used to destroy parasitic worms (helminths) including tape worms, round worms and flukes, and/or remove them from the body.
Antiemetics	Drugs that stop or prevent vomiting; these agents reduce the action of CTZ.
Antihistamine	Drug that inhibits some of the effects of histamine in the body, in particular its role in allergic reactions.
Anticholinergic	An agent inhibiting the action of acetyl choline.
Anticoagulants	An agent that prevents the clotting of blood.
Anticonvulsant	A drug that prevents or reduces the severity of fits (convlusions) in various types of epilepsy.
Antidepressant	A drug that alleviates the symptoms of depression.
Antidiuretic	(Antidiuretic hormone, ADH). A hormone released by the pituitary gland that increases the reabsorption of water by the kidney, thus preventing excessive loss of water from the body.
Antidote	A drug that counteracts the effects of a poison.
Antipruritic	An agent that relieves itching.
Antipyretic	A drug that reduces fever by lowering the body

	temperature. Several analgesic drugs have antipyretic activity.
Antiseptic	A chemical that destroys or inhibits the growth of disease causing bacteria and other microorganisms and is sufficiently non-toxic, to be applied to the skin or mucous membrane to cleanse wounds and prevent infections or to be used internally to treat infections of the intestine and bladder.
Antispasmodic	A drug that relieves spasm of smooth muscle.
Antitussive	A drug that suppresses coughing by reducing the activity of the cough centre in the brain and by depressing respiration.
Antihypertensives	Drugs that lower the blood pressure.
Antacid	An agent that reduces the stomach acidity.
Achlorhydria	Impaired secretion of gastric HCl.
Astringents	An agent used in coagulation of protein.
Anti-stomachics	Those agents which disturb the normal gastric secretion.
Bacille calmette	A strain of *Tubercle bacillus* that has lost the power
Guerin (B.C.G.)	to cause tuberculosis but retains its antigenic activity.
Bronchiolitis	Inflammation of bronchioles due to infection by bacteria or viruses.
Bronchitis	Inflammation of bronchi.
Bronchoconstrictor	A drug that causes narrowing of the air passage by producing spasm of bronchial smooth muscle.
Bronchodilator	An agent that causes widening of the air passage by producing spasm of bronchial smooth muscle.
Carcinoma	Any cancer that arises in epithelium, the tissue that lines the skin and internal organs of the body. It may occur in any tissue containing epithelial cells.
Cathartic	A drug used to stimulate or increase the frequency of bowel evacuation, or to encourage a softer or bulkier stool.

Chelating agent	A chemical compound that forms complexes by binding metal ions.
Chemotherapy	The prevention or treatment of disease by the use of chemical substances. The term is sometimes restricted to the treatment of infections diseases with antibiotics and other drugs or to the control of cancer with antimetabolites and similar drugs.
Cholengitis	Inflammation of the bile duct.
Chrysotherapy	The treatment of disease by the administration of gold or its compounds.
Cold	A widespread infectious viral disease causing inflammation of the mucous membrane of nose, throat and bronchial tubes.
Dermatitis	Inflammation of the skin caused by an outside agent.
Diabetes	Any disorder of metabolism causing excessive thirst and the production of large volumes of urine.
Diabetes insipidus	A rare metabolic disorder in which the patient produces large quantities of dilute urine and is constantly thirsty. It is due to deficiency of the pituitary hormone "vasopressin" which regulates reabsorption of water in the kidneys and is treated by administration of the hormone.
Diabetes mellitus	A disorder of carbohydrate metabolism in which sugars in the body are not oxidized to produce energy due to lack of the pancreatic hormone insulin.
Differential diagnosis	Diagnosis of a condition whose signs and/or symptoms are shared by various other conditions. For example, abdominal pain may be due to any of a large number of different disorders, which must be ruled out in arriving at a correct diagnosis.
Diphtheria	An acute highly contagious infection that is caused by the bacterium. *Corynebacterium diphtheriae*, generally affecting the throat but

	occasionally other mucous membranes and the skin.
Disinfectant	An agent that destroys or removes bacteria and other microorganisms and is used to cleanse surgical instruments and other objects, e.g. cetrimide, cresol, phenol, hexachlorophane, etc.
Disinfection	The process of eliminating infective micro-organisms from contaminated instruments, clothing or surrounding by using physical means or chemicals.
Disinfestation	The destruction of insect pests and other animal parasites.
Downs syndrome	A form of mental subnormality due to a chromosome defect.
Drug	Any substance that affects the structure or functioning of a living organism. Drugs are widely used for the prevention, diagnosis, and treatment of disease and for the relief of symptoms.
Dysaesthesiae	The abnormal and sometimes unpleasant sensations felt by a patient with partial damage to a peripheral nerve when his skin is touched. Compare paraesthesias.
Dysarthria	A speech disorder in which the pronuncation is unclear although the linguistic contact and meaning are normal.
Dysentery	An infection of the intestinal tract causing severe diarrhoea with blood and mucus and colic pain.
Dysmenorrhoea	Painful or difficult menstruation.
Dyspepsia	Disordered digestion; usually applied to pain or discomfort in the lower chest or abdomen after eating and sometimes accompanied by nausea or vomiting.
Dysphagia	A condition in which the action of swallowing is either difficult.
Dyspnoea	Difficult breathing.
Diuresis	Increased secretion of urine by kidneys.
Electro cardiogram	A recording of the electrical activity of the heart on a moving paper strip.

Emetics	An agent that causes vomiting.
Endomyocarditis	An acute or chronic inflammatory disorder of the muscle and lining membrane of the heart.
Endotoxin	A poison generally harmful to all body tissues, contained within a bacterium and release only when the bacterial cell is broken down or disintegrated.
Enterocolitis	Inflammation of the colon and small intestine.
Enuresis	The involuntary passing of urine, especially bed-wetting at night.
Enzyme	A protein that in small amounts spreads up the rate of a biological reaction without itself being used up in the reaction.
Eosinopenia	A decrease in the number of eosinophils in the blood.
Eosinophil	A variety of white blood cells distinguished by the presence of its cytoplasm of coarse granules that stain orange red with Romanowsky stains.
Eosinophilia	An increase in the number of eosinophils in the blood.
Epidermis	The outer layer of the skin.
Epilepsy	Any one of a group of disorders of brain function characterised by recurrent attacks that have a sudden onset.
Epiphora	Watering of the eye.
Erythrocyte	A blood cell containing the pigment haemoglobin.
Exoenzyme	An enzyme that acts outside the cell that produces it.
Fibrin	The final product of the process of blood coagulation, produced by the action of the enzyme thrombin on a soluble pressure fibrinogen.
Filariasis	A disease, common in the tropic and subtropics, caused by the presence in the lymph vessels of the parasitic nematode worms, *Wuchereria bancrofti*, and Brugia malay.
GABA	Gamma amino butyric acid.

Galactosaemis	An inborn inability to utilize the sugar galactose, which in consequence accumulates in the blood.
Galactose	A simple sugar and a constituent of the milk sugar lactose.
Gallstone	A hard mass compose of bile pigments, cholesterol and calcium salts, in varying proportions, than can form in the gallstones.
Gangrene	Death and decay of part of the body due to deficiency or cessation of blood sup.
Infection	Invasion of the body by harmful organisms (pathogens), such as bacteria, fungi, protozon, rickettsiae or viruses.
Inhalation	The act of breathing air into the lungs through the mouth and nose.
Inhibition	The prevention or reduction of the functioning of an organ, muscle etc.
Injection	Introduction into the body of drugs or other fluids by means of syringe.
Insufflation	The act of blowing gas or a powder such as a medication, into a body cavity.
Insomnia	Inability to fall asleep.
Jaundice	A yellowish of the skin or whites of the eyes, indicating excess bilirubin (bile pigment) in the blood.
Ketonuria	The presence of ketone (acetone) bodies in the urine.
Ketosis	Raised levels of ketone bodies in the body tissue.
Lactourisis	The presence of milk sugar (lactose) in the urine.
Laryngitis	Inflammation of the larynx and vocal cords, due to infection by bacfteria or viruses or irritation by gases, chemicals, etc.
Laxative	A drug used to stimulate or increase the frequency of bowel evacuation or to encourage or softer or bulkier stool.
Maltase	An enzyme, present in saliva and pancreatic juice.
Medicine	The science or practice of the diagnosis, treatment and prevention of disease.

Migraine	A recurrent throbbing headache that characteristically affects one side of the head.
Minimata disease	A form of mercury poisoning.
Muscle relaxant	An agent that reduces tension in muscles.
Nasal cavity	The space inside the nose that lies between the floor of the cranium and the roof of the mouth.
Nausea	The feeling that one is about to vomit.
Neutropenia	A decrease in the neutrophils in the blood.
Night blindness	The inability to see in dim light or at night.
Obesity	The condition in which excess fat has accumulated in the body, mostly in the subcutaneous tissue.
Oedema	Excessive accumulation of fluid in the body tissues. Popularly known as dropsy.
Osteomalacia	Softening of the bones caused by deficiency of vitamin D in the body.
Otorrhoea	Any discharge from the ear.
Pacemaker	A device used to produce and maintain a normal heart rate in patient who has heart block.
Paediatrics	The general medicine of childhood.
Palpitation	An awareness of the heart beat.
Paraplegia	Paralysis of both legs, usually due to disease or injury of the spiral level.
Parenteral	Administered by any way other than through the mouth.
Parkinsonism	A disorder of middle-aged and elderly people characterized by tremor, rigidity and a poverty of spontaneous movement.
Pernicious anaemia	A form of anaemia resulting from the deficiency of vitamin B_{12}.
Physician	A registered medical practitioner who specializes in the diagnosis and treatment of disease by other than surgical means.
Plague	Any epidemic disease with a high death rate.
Psoriasis	A chronic skin disease.
Rheumatic fever	An acute disease affecting mainly children and young adults that arises as a delayed complication

	of infection of the upper respiratory tract with haemolytic streptococci.
Rheumatism	Any disorder in which aches and pain affect the muscles and joints.
Rheumatoid arthritis	A form of arthritis that is the second most common rheumatic disease.
Salycylism	Poisoning due to an over dose of aspirin or other salicylate containing compounds.
Salivation	The secretion of saliva by the salivary glands of the mouth. Increased in response to the chewing action of the jaws or to thought, taste, small or sight of food.
Sarcoma	Any cancer of connective tissue.
Scabies	A skin infection caused by the itch mite, **Sarcoptes scabiei**.
Sleep	State of natural unconsciousness, during which the brain activity is not apparent but can be detected by means of an electroencephalograms.
Small pox	An acute infectious viral disease causing high fever and a rash that scars the skin.
Spinal anaesthesia	Suppression of sensation in part of the body by the injection of a local anaesthetic into the space surrounding the spiral cord.
Stomachic	An agent that stimulates the secretory activity of the stomach.
Sedative	Drugs that sedate a person so as to make him relaxed used in higher dosage, these exhibit the hypnotic effect.
Tetanus	An acute infectious disease, affecting the nervous system caused by the *Bacterium Clostririum tetani*.
Therapeutics	The branch of medicine that deals with different methods of treatment and healing (therapy), particularly the use of drugs in the cure of disease.
Thrombosis	A condition in which the blood changes from a liquid to a solid state and produces a blood clot (thrombus).

Tranquillizers	A drug that produces a calming effect, relieving anxiety and tension.
Tritanopia	A rare defect of colour vision in which affected persons are insensitive to blue light and confuse blue and green.
Tuberculosis	An infectious disease caused by bacillies *Mycobacterium tuberculosis*.
Typhoid fever	An infection of the digestive system by the bacterium *Salmonells typhi*.
Unconsciousness	A condition of being unaware of one's surrounding, as in sleep, or of being unresponsive to stimulation.
Uraemia	The presence of excessive amounts of urea and other nitrogenous waste compounds in the blood.
Vaccination	A means of producing immunity to disease by using a vaccine, or a special preparation of antigenic material, to stimulate the formation of appropriate antibodies.
Vasodilator	A drug that causes widening of the blood vessels and, therefore, an increase in blood flow.
Virulence	The disease producing (pathogenic) ability of microorganism.
Vomiting	The reflex action of ejecting the contents of the stomach through the mouth.
Wound	A break in the structure of an organ or tissue caused by an external agent. Bruises, grazes, tears, cuts, punctures and burns are all example of wounds.
Xanthinuria	The excess of the purine derivative, xanthine in the urine.
Xerophthalnia	A progressive disease of the eye due to deficiency of vitamin A.
Yellow fever	An infectious disease caused by an arbovirus, occurring in tropical Africa and the northern regions of South America.
Yawning	A reflex action in wich the mouth is opened wide and air is drawn into the lungs then slowly released. It is a result of drowsiness, fatigue or boredom.

Zollinger-Ellison syndrome	A disorder in which there is an excessive secretion of gastric juice due to high level of circulating gastrin.
Zymolysis	The process of fermentation or digestion by an enzyme.
Zymotic disease	An old name for a contagious disease which was formerly thought to develop within the body following infection in a process similar to the fermentation and growth of yeast.

COMMONLY USED LATIN ABBREVIATION

Abbreviation	*Full latin words*	*English translations*
ad	Ad	Up to, to
ad lib.	Ad libitum	As needed, at pleasure
agit	Agita	Shake
All hor	Alterni horis	Alternate hour
aa	Ana	Of each
a.c.	Ante Cibos	Before meal
aq. dist.	Aqua distillata	Distilled water
b.i.d.	Bis in die	Twice daily
cap.	Capiat	Take
Chart	Charta	Paper
Coch. amp.	Cochleare amplum	Table spoonful
Coch. mag.	Cochleare magnum	Table spoonful
Coch. parv.	Cochleare parvum	Tea spoonful
Collum.	Collunarium	Nose wash
Collut	Collutorium	Mouth wash
Collyr.	Collyrium	Eye wash
$\bar{c}$	Cum	With
d.t.d.	Denture tales doses	Give of such doses
e.m.p.	Ex modo prescripto	In the prescribed manner
F, Ft	Fiat	Make
gtt.	Gutta	Drop
h.s.	Hora somni	Bed time
liq.	Liquor	Solution

man.	Mane	Morning
M.	Misc.	Mix
m. dict.	Mode dictu	As directed
mor. dict	More dictu	As directed
omn.	Omni.	Every
p.o.	per os	Orally, by mouth
p.c.	post cibos	After meals
p.r.n.	Pro re nata	When needed
pulv.	Pulvis	Powder
q.d.	Quanque die	Every day
q.m.	Quaque manc	Every morning
q.n.	Quaque nocte	Every night
q.r.	Quantitum rectum	The quantity is correct
q.i.	Quantitum sufficit	A sufficient quantity
q.i.d.	Quarter in die	Four times a day
R	Recipe	Take, thou take, you take
s.a.	Secundum artem	According to the art, pharmaceutically
s.s.	semi	Half
sig.	Signa	Write
$\bar{s}$	Sine	Without
s.o.s.	S. opus sit	When need arises
stat.	Statim	Immediately
t.i.d.	Ter in die	Three times
ung.	Ouguentum	Ointment
ut. dict.	Ut. dictum	As directed

20
Chapter

Diseases : Manifestation and Pathophysiology

This chapter provides a knowledge regarding some major diseases. It needs the understanding of the following few terms :

1. **Etiology :** It deals with identification of causative agents which provoke a particular disease. For example *Mycobacterium tuberculosis* is the etiologic agent for tuberculosis. Other secondary etiologic factors include the nutritional one, age and sanitation conditions.
2. **Pathogenesis :** Pathogenesis of disease refers to the development or evolution of diseases, e.g. pathogenesis of tuberculosis indicates how the *Mycobacterium tuberculosis*, causative organism, enters in the body and develops the tuberculosis.
3. **Manifestation :** These are various changes, occur during the disease process.
4. **Lesion :** It is a recognizable structural changes, observed during the development of disease.
5. **Signs and symptoms :** Symptoms are the subjective feelings, reported by the diseased person to a doctor while signs are recognizable changes. Nausea, malaise and pain are symptoms while fever and rashes on skin are signs of the disease.
6. **Sequel :** The outcome of a disease is called sequel. Formation of scar due to inflammation is the sequel of that disease process.
7. **Complication of a disease :** It is a separate process that may develop secondary due to some changes produced in the main disease. *Bacterial pneumonia* may be a complication of viral infection of the respiratory tract.

TUBERCULOSIS

Tuberculosis is a bacterial infection. It usually involves the lungs but may affect any organ or tissue in the body.

Etiology : *Mycobacterium tuberculosis* is rod-shaped micro-organism that requires oxygen tension for optimum growth and produces no toxin. *M. tuberculosis hominies* is responsible for most cases of infection. Transmission is usually directed by inhalation of airborne organisms or by exposure to contaminated patient secretion. Oropharyngeal and intestinal tuberculosis are occurred by drinking milk contaminated with *Mycobacterium bovis*.

Pathophysiology : *Tubercle bacilli* are inhaled and deposited in peripheral alveoli throughout the lung. This is the primary tuberculosis. From the lungs, infection spread throughout the body by lymphatic system. The *Tubercle bacilli* is deposited in kidney, growing ends of bone and other areas of high oxygen tension. Cellular immunity involving lymphocytes, macrophages develops and prevents its spread. During caseation, cytotoxic material is released from lymphocytes which destroys the bacilli as well as surrounding tissues. The site then heals by resolution, fibrosis and calcification. The healed lesion still contains viable *Tubercle bacilli*. Organisms may remain inactive for the life of the host or they may be reactivated. Reactivation usually occurs under circumstance of decreased immunity as in malnutrition, underlying disease, old age or treatment with corticosteroid.

Signs and Symptoms

Stage I : The initial infection or primary tuberculosis usually does not provide many signs or symptoms. The incubation period is 4 to 8 weeks. Mild fever and malaise may occur as tuberculin hypersensitivity develops.

Stage II : Pulmonary tuberculosis usually occurs after a period of dormancy in previously infected individual. Fever to 40°C may occur in late afternoon or evening. Night sweats are common. General malaise, fatigue, irritability and weight loss may occur. A cough, particularly early in the morning and production of yellow sputum that may be blood streaked is common. Blood is present due to ulceration of bronchial mucosa. Massive haemorrhage can occur if a pulmonary artery in a tuberculous cavity ruptures. Death may occur from obstruction of airflow.

Spreads of pulmonary tuberculosis into pleura results in pleuritic chest pain and the formation of pleural effusion as part of the inflammatory reaction. The presence of large pleural effusion cause dyspnoea.

Stage III : Military tuberculosis is a massive dissemination of *Tubercle bacilli* throughout the body. Lesion are also found in addition to lungs in the liver, spleen, bone marrow and other organs which do not have high oxygen tension. The signs and symptoms are nonspecific and include dyspnoea, weight loss, weakness, fever, night sweats and gastrointestinal disturbances. Death is certain unless appropriate treatment is introduced.

HEPATITIS

Hepatitis is a term used by the pathologist to describe the presence of inflammation in the liver. Hepatitis may be caused by a large number of infectious organism, therapeutic agents and toxins. Only viral hepatitis due to hepatotropic viruses is discussed here.

Etiology

The known causative hepatotropic viruses are :

Hepatitis A virus, Hepatitis B virus, the Hepatitis B associated delta virus (Hepatitis D virus), Hepatitis C virus, Hepatitis E virus, the last two referred formerly to as non-A and non-B Hepatitus viruses. All these viruses cause acute hepatitis, the epidemology, the spectrum of liver injury and the incidence of chronicity vary with pathogens.

Hepatitis A virus (HAV) is a small, non-enveloped RNA virus that causes a benign, acute, self limited disorder that does not lead chronicity. Hepatitis A was formerly referred to as "infectious hepatitis" or short incubation hepatitis because incubation period is small, only 15 to 45 days.

Hepatitis B virus (HBV) is DNA virus, formerly known as "serum hepatitis" have a long incubation period, usually occurs 30 days to 6 months after exposure to infected blood or serum.

Pathology

In the Hepatitis B, virus replicates in the liver cell and it or its fragments are incorporated into liver cell membrane. Humeral antibodies IgG and IgM are formed against the viruses. Antibodies attack the 'foreign' plasma membranes. Cellular immunity is involved in the liver damage. Circulating immune complexes and complement activation are responsible for the manifestation such as vasculitis and polyarthrites.

Thus, the consequences of Hepatitis B are largely due to immune response to infection rather than the cytotoxicity of the virus. The pathophysiology of other forms of viral hepatitis is less understood.

Signs and Symptoms

In hepatitis following symptoms appear :

(i) There may be anorexia, nausea, vomiting changes in the smell and taste, fatigue, malaise, arthralgias, myalgias, headache photophobia, pharyngitis, cough and fever. These symptoms appear 1 to 2 weeks before onset of jaundice.

(ii) Urine becomes a dark in colour due to bilirubinenia and clay coloured stools may occur 1 to 5 days before jaundice.

(iii) Liver is enlarged and becomes tender. There may be right upper quadrant pain.

(iv) The recovery phase lasts from 2 to 14 weeks but longer period in Hepatitis B. Laboratory abnormalities disappear in 3 to 4 months.

(v) Several liver cell enzymes including serum amino transferases increase which mark the onset of jaundice. Jaundice is visible in the skin and sclera when serum bilirubin level exceeds 2.5 mg/100 ml. Jaundice is maximum between 1st and 2nd week but then decreases. Usually jaundice last in 6 to 8 weeks.

Serological markers are used to distinguish between the different types of viral hepatitis. In Hepatitis A, there is sharp rise in IgM anti HAV and a gradual but lasting rise in IgG anti HAV. Hepatitis B is characterized by sharp rise in surface antigen, HBsAg. There are no serological markers for Hepatitis C and Hepatitis E. The diagnosis is made on the basis of compatible clinical features and the absence of serological markers of Hepatitis A and Hepatitis B.

RHEUMATOID ARTHRITIS (RA)

Rheumatoid arthritis is a systemic, chronic, inflammatory disease that affects principally the joints and sometimes many other organs and tissue throughout the body as well.

Etiology

The etiology etiology of RA is not clear. There is genetic predisposition to RA and joint inflammation in immunologically mediated. Some unknown environmental factors may play a role in development of RA.

Phathophysiology

Autoimmunity is considered to by primary abnormality in RA. Autoantibodies are found against all immunoglobins (IgM, IgG and IgA). They are found to be present in serum and synovial fluids. These antibodies are called rheumatoid factor (RF). Synovial fluid IgG rheumatoid factors self associate (IgG – anti-IgG) to form immune complexes that activate complement, attract polymorphonuclear leucocytes and lead to tissue injury. These rheumatoid factor amplify joint inflammation.

Signs and Symptoms

The rheumatoid arthritis first appear insidiously with aching and stiffness of the joints particularly in the morning. As the disease progresses, the joints become enlarged and motion is limited. Joint stiffness particularly after a prolonged period of rest is major complaint with RA. The commonly affected joints are hand, feet, shoulders, knees, elbows, ankles and wrist. Muscle weakness and atrophy often augment the severity of the joint disease. Flexion contractures and ankylosis develop as the disease progresses. The fingers may become virtually immobilized in claw-like position with ulnar deviation. At this stage of the disease, anemia is common.

After 15 to 20 years, the majority of patients become permanently and severely crippled.

CARDIOVASCULAR DISEASES

Atherosclerosis

The most common form of heart disease is caused by atherosclerosis. It is generally referred to as coronary heart disease or hardening and/or thickening of the arteries. Atherosclerosis involves the slow buildup of deposits of fatty substances, cholesterol, body cellular waste products, calcium and fibrin (a clotting material in the blood) in the inside lining of an artery. The buildup that results (referred to as plaque) can partially or totally block the flow of blood through the artery. This can lead to the formation of a blood clot (thrombus) on the surface of the plaque. If either of these events occurs and blocks the entire artery, a heart attack or stroke may result.

Etiology

Although the terms are used interchangeably, atherosclerosis (or "hardening of the arteries") is one type of arteriosclerosis. Artheriosclerosis is actually a generic term for a number of diseases in which the arterial wall becomes thickened and loses elasticity. The term atherosclerosis is derived from combing the Greek words athero (paste) and sclerosis (hardness). Atherosclerosis involves a process that causes a build-up of deposits on artery walls called plaque. Typically, the deposits occur in the tunica intima (the innermost layer of a blood vellel) of large and medium-sized arteries. The plaques contain fatty substances, cholesterol, cellular waste products, fibrin found in blood, and calcium. Plaque can become large enough to partially or totally block the flow of blood through an artery. A build-up of plaque or a rupture occurring within the plaque can result in a blood clot. The dislodged plaque material can travel to other parts of the body (e.g. brain, heart, kidneys and legs), resulting in serious injury to tissues and principally by blocking blood flow through smaller arteries. Atherosclerosis is a progressive, complex disease often associated with the ageing process, but for some it starts much earlier in life.

Pathophysiology

The mechanism for the development of atherosclerosis is poorly understood. Probably lesions are developed due to increased stress associated with increased blood pressure and turbulent blood flow. Platelet aggregation occurs in lesion of inner layer of arterial wall (intima). This condition is known as *atheroma*. These changes may induce smooth muscle proliferation along with lipid accumulation. Finally fibrosis, calcification, haemorrhage, ulceration and thrombosis develop, causing reduction in blood flow due to lumen narrowing.

Signs and Symptoms

The signs and symptoms of atherosclerosis disease depend on the location and degree of impairment of blood flow to an organ.

In severe case, it may cause angina pectoris, myocardial, infarction, cerebrovascular accident, thrombosis, ischemic renal disease, peripheral vascular disease and even death.

There may be pain in legs at night when blood does not flow due to gravity, weakness of muscle, loss of pulses in the feet, extreme sensitivity to cold and eventually dry gangrene. Atherosclerosis of the mesenteric velles may cause abdominal pain, weight loss and diarrhoea. Thrombosis of these vessel causes bowel infarction.

Angina Pectoris

Angina Pectoris is not a disease but a symptom of myocardial ischemia. It develops as a result of an imbalance between the oxygen supply and the oxygen demand of the myocardium.

Pathophysiology

In angina, the capacity of oxygen supply is limited. Oxygen consumption of the myocardium rises with increasing heart size, heart rate, systemic blood pressure and myocardial contractility (velocity at which the muscle shortens). The last three stages are increased by more sympathetic activity. Tachycardia increases the total systolic fraction of cardiac cycle and contractility of the myocardium. Exercise, anaemia and hyperthyroidism also increase myocardial oxygen requirement.

Sign and Symptoms

Angina pectoris is usually felt by tightness in the chest. It is usually induced by exertion and relieved by rest, lasting only a few minutes. Some patients feel the pain in chest during some activity, e.g. running, walking (*Angina of efforts*). *Angina at rest* is characterized by chest pain at rest. Rarely, pain may come as a result of coronary arterial spasm.

Cardiac Arrythmia

It is an irregularity in the heart beat.

Pathophysiology

The pathophysiological mechanism responsible for arrythmia is not clearly understood. It is generally accepted that arrythmia may arise either due to disorder of impulse formation or disorders of impulse conduction.

Tachycardia due to disturbed impulse formation is associated with irregular and rhythmic discharge from ectopic pacemaker activity in other areas of the myocardium. The atrial arrythmias occur due to discharge of impulses from ectopic pacemaker.

Disorders of impulse conduction is more common mechanism of arrythmias. Some area of myocardium has areas of depressed function with prolonged refractory periods. Due to this, an impulse approaching such an area would be diverted to adjacent excitable tissue. It is possible that the same impulse, after taking a circular route through normal tissue, will again reach the depressed area which by then become excitable. Upon traversing it, the excitatory process is free to re-enter normal region and therapy restimulate the chamber or entire heart. Repetition of this cycle is possible and so produce an ectopic tachycardia.

Signs and Symptoms

Different types of arrythmias are mentioned here :

(i) *Sinus bradycardia* : Heart rate is less than 60 beats per minute with the impulse originating in the sinus node. Sinus bradycardia occurs in individuals having intracerebral pressure, hypothyroidism or in patient with SA node dysfunction.

(ii) Sinus arrest refers to total cessation of sinus node activity.

(iii) Sinus arrythmia is not an arrythmia but a normal change in heart rate that occurs with respiration. Heart rate increases during inspiration and decreases during expiration.

(iv) *Sinus tachycardia* : In this, there is a heart rate greater than 100 beats per minute which may be due to anxiety, fever, anaemia, blood loss, hypoxemia and electrolyte disturbances.

(v) *Atrial flutter* : It is a regular thythm with an average atrial rate of 300 beat/minute. The ventricle beat is 75 to 150 beat/minute which reflect AV block. It occurs in patients with ischemic heart disease.

(vi) *Atrial fibrillation* : It is an arrythmia in which arteries do not contract so cardiac output is decreased and symptoms of congestive heart failure may appear. It may occur in digitalis intoxication.

Myocardial Infarction

This is myocardial necrosis occurring as a result of a critical imbalance between coronary blood supply and myocardial demand.

It is usually due to the formation of occlusive thrombus at the site of rupture of an atheromatous plaque in a coronary artery. Myocardial infarction may occur in any location in the left or right ventricle depending on which coronary artery is occluted.

Signs and Symptoms

There is pain like an angina but it is more persistent and more severe. It lasts for 30 minutes to many hours. Other symptoms include anxiety, vomiting, sweating, tachycardia, low systolic pressure and reduced pulse pressure.

Hypertension

Hypertension means abnormally elevated blood pressure. It is not a disease but is a physical finding. Hypertension is said where there is sustained diastolic pressure greater than 90 mmHg or sustained systolic pressure in excess of 140 mmHg. Clinical consequences are different in diastolic and systolic hypertension.

Etiology

Nearly 10 to 20% cases of hypertension have some reasons and so these are called *secondary hypertension*. It includes renal disease and endocrine disorders. The remaining 80 to 90% cases of hypertension have no definite cause and so called idiopathic, primary or essential. It is due to abnormalities in physiological regulatory system, e.g. genetic defect in renal sodium excretion, defect in sodium/calcium transport in vascular smooth muscle or increase release of vasoconstrictor agent like renin and catecholamine. Systolic hypertension also occurs in conditions of increased cardiac output such as anemia, fever, beriberi, aortic valve insufficiency and thyrotoxicosis.

Pathophysiology

Hypertension is a main risk factor for atherosclerosis and cardiovascular complications such as congestive heart failure, myocardial infarction and angina pectoris. Sustained hypertension causes damage in target organs – the eyes, brain, heart and kidneys.

Hypertensive retinopathy leads to visual disturbances. Damage to brain due to hypertension includes cerebral edema, thrombosis and haemorrhage.

The heart compensates for the increased work imposed by the increased afterload with left ventricular hypertrophy. Left ventricular function deteriorates, chamber dilates and left ventricular failure occurs.

Hypertension accelerates coronary atherosclerotic heart disease and increases myocardial oxygen consumption. Angina pectoris and myocardial infarction are more common in hypertensive patients.

Hypertension causes fibrin deposition in glomeruli and muscular hypertrophy of afferent arterioles. There may be development of fibrinoid necrosis in the afferent arterioles due to increased permeability to fibrinogen and other plasma protein followed by platelet deposition. Malignant hypertension accelerates kidney damage which leads to renal failure.

Signs and Symptoms

Hypertension causes no signs or symptoms unless the B.P. is very high. The signs and symptoms of essential hypertension are secondary to target organ damage.

Retinopathy causes scotomas, blurred vision and finally blindness.

Brain damage may cause dizziness, headache, vertigo, tinnitus, convulsions and coma.

Damage to heart results in angina pectoris or the signs and symptoms of chronic heart failure or myocardial infarction.

Renal failure may also occur.

Epilepsy

Epilepsy is a group of disorders in which there are recurrent episodes of altered cerebral function with paroxysmal excessive and hyperchronous discharge of cerebral neurones. The clinical accompaniments of these episodes-seizures vary in manifestation from brief lapses of awareness to prolonged of unconsciousness, limb jerking and incontinence.

Etiology

Many diseases may cause seizures but it is not epilepsy. Diseases involving central nervous system such as brain tumours, cerebral vascular accidents, meningitis, lipid storage diseases and cerebral injuries may cause epilepsy. Many cases of epilepsy are idiopathic in origin of which cause is unidentifiable.

Pathophysiology

The convulsion results from sudden excessive neuronal discharges in a normal or diseased cortex. The reason of excessive discharge is unknown but there are two theory to explain this.

One theory states that diencephalic nerves normally exerts a constant restraining influence on cortical neurons preventing excessive discharge. In epilepsy, the neurons are deafferented, supersensitive and susceptible to activation by various stimuli.

Another theory states that there is a decreased amount of gamma aminobutyric acid (GABA) which is one of the inhibitory transmitter in the brain.

The excessive disorderly neuron discharge effects the entire brain, which results in loss of consciousness and convulsive movements.

Signs and Symptoms

The signs and symptoms of epilepsy depend on the type of epilepsy. It is generally classified as generalized of partial.

Generalized Seizures

They affect the entire cerebral cortex and are of two type :

(i) *Grand mal epilepsy* : It is characterized by sudden loss of consciousness, a cry, falling and clinic movements of muscles. The patient may be unconscious for as long as 30 minutes.

(ii) *Petilmal epilepsy* : There is loss of consciousness for few seconds. The patient has a blank expression and may blink the eyelids or jerk the arm.

Partial Seizures

They start from one side of brain and are of two types :

(i) Focal epilepsy, also called partial epilepsy, which begins with twitching of the fingers of one hand, the face or one foot. The movement then spreads to other muscles on the same side of body. Later on, it may become generalized.

(ii) Psychomotor epilepsy is often associated with a lesion in the temporal lobe. The patient remain conscious, perform work normally but may not able to respond to question or command. This type of seizure may last for hours.

Diabetes Mellitus

Diabetes mellitus is a chronic disorder of carbohydrate, fat and protein metabolism. A defective or deficient insulin secretary response causes the impaired carbohydrate metabolism which results in hypoglycemia.

Etiology

Primary diabetes mellitus, also called idiopathic diabetes mellitus is inherited, the cause of this unknown. This can be basically divided into two variants that differs in their pattern of inheritance, insulin response and origins.

(i) The first is insulin dependent diabetes mellitus (IDDM) also called Type I diabetes, previously known as juvenile onset. This variant accounts for 10 to 20% of all cases of idiopathic diabetes.

(ii) The remaining 80 to 90% of patients have the second variant, non-insulin dependent diabetes mellitus (NIDDM), also called Type II diabetes.

Secondary diabetes includes hypoglycemia associated with identifiable causc in which destruction of pancreatic islets is induced by inflammatory pancreatic disease, surgery, tumors, certain drugs and iron overload (hemochromatosis).

Pathophysiology

In deficient insulin, glucose is not utilized by the liver, which results in hypoglycemia.

Insulin facilitates the entry of glucose into cells and stimulates protein synthesis. The lack of glucose in muscle cells leads to glycogenolysis and release of amino acid for gluconeogenesis.

Lack of insulin and glucose in adipose tissues cause the impaired triglyceride synthesis and release of free fatty acids.

The liver metabolizes free fatty acid to ketones which are used by the muscles to limited extent for energy.

Hypoglycemia results in *glucosuria* when the serum level of glucose exceeds the renal threshold for reabsorption of glucose. Glucosuria results in *polyuria* due to osmotic diuresis. It may result in dehydration. Excess ketone bodies are excreted in the urine as strong acids which results in urinary loss of bicarbonate and potassium which results in dehydration.

Glycoprotein is deposited in the capillaries due to hypoglycemia. Glucose is metabolised to sorbitol by aldose reductase in hyperglycemia which produces cataracts and neuropathy.

Sign and Symptoms

On set of Type I diabetes is sudden and characterized by polyuria, weight loss, decreased muscle strength and irritability.

Ketoacidosis is common in Type I diabetes. Other Symptoms of diabetes mellitus include tingling, numbness in the feet, and slow healing of skin infections.

After a long period, diabetics often develops kidney failure, lesions of the eyes and atrophy of the peripheral nerves.

PEPTIC ULCER

It can be defined as 'hole in the mucosa' of any portion of gastrointestinal tract exposed to acid-pepsin secretion. Duodenal ulcers and gastric ulcers are the main types of peptic ulcers.

Duodenal Ulcer

Among ulcers 80% ulceration is of *duodenal ulcer*.

Pathophysiology

The pathogenesis of duodenal ulcer is manifactorial. This type of ulcer never occur in absence of gastric acid. The hypersecretion of acid may be due to an increased parietal cell mass, excessive gastric release during meals, enhanced sensitivity of gastric or to other factors. Some patients have an increased rate of gastric emptying of acid. Duodenal ulcer occurs more frequently in patients with hyperparathyriodism, alcoholic cirrhosis and rheumatoid arthritis.

Sign and Symptoms

Duodenal ulcer is characterized by remission and exacerbations. It starts with acute inflammation of duodenal mucosa. There is a burning pain in the mid-epigastrium which is relieved by ingestion of food or antacid. The pain begins about 2 hours after a meal, may awaken the patients between midnight and 3.00 a.m. but almost never present before breakfast. The patient often gains weight because eating relieves the pain. These may be mild tenderness in the mild-epigastrium and iron deficiency anaemia. The ulcer may perforate into the peritoneal cavity resulting in peritonitis and sepsis.

Gastric ulcer : It occurs in the stomach. It is less common than duodenal ulcer.

Pathophysiology

It never occur in absence of acid. Sometimes patients with gastric ulcer secrete less acid that do the normal people. Pathogenesis of gastric ulcer includes gastric hypomotility, abnormalities in mucosa, blood flow and alteration in gastric barrier which allow the back diffusion of hydrogen ions into the mucosa. Cigarette smoking and aspirin ingestion increase the risk of developing gastric ulcer disease.

Signs and Symptoms

There is a burning pain in gastric ulcer which is less localized than duodenal ulcer pain. This pain is reduced after ingestion of food. The pain in gastric ulcer rarely occurs in night. Gastric ulcer complication includes peritonitis, sepsis and pancreatitis.

AIDS

Acquired immune deficiency syndrome or **acquired immunodeficiency syndrome (AIDS** or **Aids)** is a set of symptoms and infections resulting from the damage to the human immune system caused by the Human Immunodeficiency Virus (HIV). This condition progressively reduces the effectiveness of the immune system and leaves individuals susceptible to opportunistic infections and tumors.

Etiology

HIV is transmitted through direct contact of a mucous membrane or the bloodstream with a bodily fluid containing HIV, such as blood, semen, vaginal fluid, preseminal fluid, and breast milk. This transmission can involve anal, vaginal or oral sex, blood transfusion, contaminated hypodermic needles, exchange between mother and baby during pregnancy, childbirth, or breastfeeding, or other exposure to one of the above bodily fluids.

Signs and Symptoms

The symptoms of AIDS are primarily the result of conditions that do not normally develop in individuals with healthy immune system. Most of the conditions are infections caused by bacteria, viruses, fungi and parasites that are normally controlled by the elements of the immune system that HIV damages. Early signs and symptoms of HIV can include candidiasis, lymphadenopathy, cervical carcinoma, herpes zoster and peripheral neuropathy. Late signs and symptoms of HIV and AIDS defining illnesses can include the development of life-threatening infections and malignancies. Additionally, people with AIDS often have systemic symptoms of infection like fevers, sweats (particularly at night), swollen glands, chills, weakness and weight loss.

Pathophysiology

There are two types of HIV (HIV-1 and HIV-2) that cause AIDS. The causative agent of HIV infection in most of the world is HIV-1, HIV-2 is seen for the most part in Africa. HIV is a retrovirus, which means it carries genetic information in RNA as opposed to DNA. HIV cannot replicate without a host. HIV targets specialized white blood cells of the immune system called $CD^{4+}T^{-}$ lymphocytes (T-cells). It infects the T-cell by binding the CD^{4+} receptor site of the cell. An enzyme called reverse transcriptase converts the HIV, RNA to DNA, thus damaging the CD^{4+} T-cell. The T-cell is then stimulated to reproduce, however, the DNA has been changed in the cell, so it now produces new HIV viral particles called virons. The HIV infected T^{+} cell produces more than 30,000 virons. Virons released from the infected T-cell travel to normal T-cells infecting them and producing more HIV virons. The number of normally functioning T-cells decrease rapidly, weakening the immune system. As CD^{4+} T-cells are depleted, viral levels rise until there are few uninfected T-cells left.

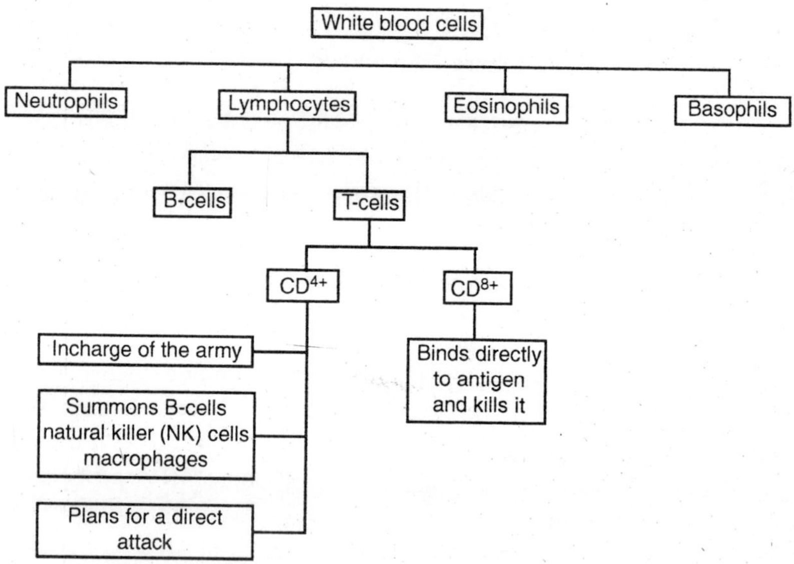

Fig. 19.1. Immune response shown by white blood cells.

21

Chapter

Physiological Parameters

Human body consists of various complex systems which may be further divided into sub-systems. Health depends on proper functioning of these systems. Disease occurs if any system does not function in a proper way and it may be reflected by deviation in some physiological parameters. Some important parameters together with their clinical significance are discussed in this chapter.

BLOOD EXAMINATION

1. **Haemoglobin value :** Haemoglobin is the red pigment of blood. It is composed of globin (96%) and haem, the iron containing pigment (4%). Haemoglobin concentration is expressed in g %.

   Normal range

   Male 15.5 ± 2.5 g %

   Female 14 ± 2.5 g %

   Infants upto 18 g %

   Clinical significance : Haemoglobin value below normal range causes anaemia and leukemias. This value rises above normal range in dehydration and polycythemia.

2. **Cell counts :** Normally blood contains three types of cells :

   (i) Red blood corpuscles (RBC)

   (ii) White blood corpuscles (WBC)

   (iii) Platelets.

   These are expressed as number of cells per cubic millimeter.

(i) Red Blood Corpuscles, Count RBC

The red are most numerous cells in the blood and contain a haemoglobin which give them their red colour. The RBC are formed in the red bone marrow.

Normal range :

Male	4.5 to 5.5 million/mm^3
Female	3.5 to 5.5 million/mm^3
Children	4 to 5.5 million/mm^3

Clinical significance

Increased RBC number above normal range indicates heart ailment, polycythaemia, cholera while while decreased number indicates the anaemia.

Hematocrit (Hct) value

It directly measure the RBC mass. It is important in determination of anemia or polycythemia. It is 40-54% in adult males and 37-47% for adult females.

(ii) Total White Blood Corpuscles (WBC) Count

WBC, also called leucocytes, are colourless cells, containing nuclei. They are little larger in size than RBC but less in number. Total leukocyte count (TLC) varies between 4000 and 11000 per cubic millimeter but 8000 per mm^3 is a normal average value.

Clinical Significance

High TLC value (leucocytosis) is found in appendicites, leukemia, pneumonia, diptheriae, small pox, tonsilitis, meningitis, rheumatic fever, etc.

Low TLC value (leucopenia) is found in typhoid, hepatitis, influenza, measles, paratyphoid and agranulocytosis.

(iii) Differential Leucocyte Count (DLC)

Various types of white blood cells are as follows :

Neutrophils	60 to 70%
Eosinophils	1 to 4%
Basophils	0 to 1%
Monocytes	5 to 10%
Lymphocytes	25 to 30%

Clinical Significance

Both TLC and DLC are helpful in detecting infectious disease.

A high neutrophil count indicates the severe infection. Eosinophils are high in worm infestation and allergic conditions. Basophils increase in granulocytic leukemia. Lymphocyte number is high in whooping cough. Monocytes increase in bacterial infection/malaria and monocytic leukemia.

(iv) Erythrocyte Sedimentation Rate (ESR)

It is the at which erythrocyte sedimentation takes place on their own weight when anticoagulant blood is held in a vertical column. It is expressed as the fall of RBC's in mm at the end of first hour.

Normal range :

(a) Western green's method :

Male	0-5 mm at the end of first hour
Female	0-7 mm at the end of first hour

(b) Wintrobe's methods :

Male	0-9 mm at the end of first hour
Female	0-20 mm at the end of first hour

Clinical Significance

High ESR value is found in rheumatic fever, rheumatoid arthritis, tuberculosis, allergy, syphilis, cancer, pneumonia and malignant tumors.

(v) Coagulation Time/Clotting Time of Blood

It is the time required by the blood to clot.

Normal range

Capillary blood methods :

(a) Slide method	2-6 minutes
(b) Capillary tube method	2-6 minutes

Venous blood methods

(a) Howell method	0 to 30 minutes
(b) Lee and White method	5 to 15 minutes

Clinical Significance

Clotting time is more in haemophilia, vitamin K deficiency, obstructive jaundice, dicoumarol therapy, heparin therapy, pneumonia and leukemia.

(vi) Blood Sugar

Normal range of blood sugar level is 80-120 mg/100 ml. The excess of this level is detected in hyperglycaemia and below this level is found hypoglycaemia.

Clinical Significance

Hyperglycaemia leads to diabetes in which sugar level may rise up to 500 mg/100 ml. Sometime it may cross this level also, which causes the coma. Hyperglycaemia also occurs in adrenal cortical hyper activity and obesity. Hypoglycaemia may occur in insulin overdosage, pancreatic tumour adrenal cortical insufficiency and hypopitutarism.

Glucose Tolerance Test

The normal and diabetic response using an oral glucose (75 g) are mentioned below :

	Whole blood glucose concentration (m mol/l)	
	Normal	Diabetic
Fasting	< 6.1 (5-6)	≥ 7.8 (6.7)
2 hours after glucose	< 6.9 (6.7)	≥ 11.1 (10.0)

(vii) Blood Cholesterol

Normal values of total cholesterol are as follows :

Neonates	45-100 mg %
20-30 years	145-275 mg %
30-40	169-295 mg %
40-50	170-315 mg %
Above 50 years	175-350 mg %

Clinical Significance

Cholesterol level rises in diabetes mellitus, obstructive jaundice, obesity, myxedema, xanthomatous disorders and familial hyperlipoproteinemias.

(viii) Blood Uric Acid

Normal value is 2-6 mg/100 ml. In females the normal value is slightly lower.

(ix) Blood Urea Nitrogen (BUN)

It is measure of amount of nitrogen in the blood that come from urea.

Normal human blood contain 7-25 mg of uea nitrogen per 100 ml. The elevation lvel indicates impaired renal function.

Clinical Significance

Uric acid level rises in gout, excessive dietary purines, psoriasis and renal failure.

Heart Rate

It is a pulse rate per minute. Normal value of heart rate at different age is as follows :

Foetus	140-150/minute
Neonatal	130-140/minute
One year	115-130/minute
2-3 year	100-115/minute
7-14 year	80-90/minute
Over 15 years	70-80/minute

(x) Serum Creatinine

It is breakdown product of creatine phosphate in muscle. The typical reference range for women 0.5 to 1.0 mg/dL and for men 0.7 to 1.2 mg/dL. A rising creatinine level indicates kidney damage.

Clinical Significance

Heat rate reflects the condition of heart directly and blood pressure indirectly. Heart rate increases in excitement, fever and muscular exercise.

STOOL EXAMINATION

The average healthy adults defecate from two-three times a day to three times a week common pattern is once a day. The stool tends to be soft and bulky depending on a diet. Two-thirds of the stool weight is attributable to its water content. The normal brown colour is of still undetermined origin. The odour is due to presence of indole and scatole, formed by microbes from tryptophan.

Clinical Significance

A simple inspection of faces lead to a diagnosis of parasitic infestation (Ascan's lumbricoids, talnia, sps. etc), obstructive jaundice, diarrhoea, dysentery or ulcerative colitis or gastro-intestinal tract bleeding. Generally macroscopic and microscopic examinations are done.

Macroscopic Examination

In this test, the form, consistency and colour of stool are observed.

Type of stool	*Probable reason*
Watery stool	Diarrhoea
Large amount of mushy, four smelling, gray stool which float on water	Steatorrhoea
Little firm, spherical masses	Constipation
Narrow ribbon like stool	Spastic bowel or rectal narrowing
Clay coloured	Obstructive jaundice
Reddish stool	Blood from lower gastro-intestinal tract
Black, tarry stool	Bleeding from upper gastro-intestinal tract, iron, bismuth or charcoal consumption
Green stool	Ingestion of spinach other green vegetables, calomel, presence of biliveridin seen in patient taking antibiotics orally
Mucousy stool	Chronic ulcerative colitis and chronic bacillary dysentery
Microscopic examination	
Cells	RBC's, mucous and pus cells indicate amoebic dysentery and macrophages, pus, cells indicate bacillary dysentery
Parasites and eggs	Protozoans : *Entamoeba histolytica* and *Entamoeba coli, Trichomonas hominis, Giardia lambia* (Giardiasis), *Balantidium coli* (Balantidiasis) Helminthes : Eggs are seen in helminthes infestation

URINE EXAMINATION

Normal urine is a clear, yellow or amber coloured fluid having a specific gravity varying between 1.003 to 1.030. It is usually slightly acidic and has a faintly aromatic odour. It consists of 96% water and 4% solid content. Solid contents include urea, creatinine, uric acid, iron, chlorides, sodium, calcium and phosphate.

Urine examination is also divided into physical and chemical examination.

Physical Examination

Volume	1200-2000 ml	It is increased in polyuria and decreased in renal disease
Specific gravity	1.005-1.025	Specific gravity is high in diabetes and low in nephritis

Colour

Milky	Genito-urinary tract disease
Orange	Urobilinogenuria
Red	Haematuria
Greenish	Jaundice

Chemical Examination

pH	4.8-7.5 with	pH is less than 4.8 in diabetes, staria-tion and febrile illness in children
Protein	Abnormal constituent (Proteinuria)	Nephritis Nephrosis Pregnancy
Sugar	Abnormal constituent (Hyperglycemic)	Diabetes, Pancreatic disease, CNS dysfunction
Bile pigment	Abnormal constituent	Jaundice
Ketone bodies		
Acetone, aceto-acetic acid and β-hydroxybutyric acid)	Abnormal constituent Vomiting	Diabetes, Cachexia, Post anaesthesia
Blood cells	Abnormal constituent	Haematuria
Calcium	Abnormal constituent	Hyperparathyroidism

SPUTUM EXAMINATION

Tracheobronchial secretions are often collectively referred to as sputum. Sputum is constituted by plasma, water, electrolytes and mucin. As it comes out, it is contaminated by nasal and salivary secretion and normal bacterial flora of the oral cavity. Under appropriate immunologic or inflammatory stimulus, mast cells, eosinophils and plasma cells may contribute to the secretions. Chemical composition reveals sputums is

95% water and only 5% solids. The solid content increases with inflammation.

It is divided into two healing—Macroscopic and microscopic examinations.

Macroscopic Examination

1. *Volume*, 24 hour volume of sputum is measured.
2. *Consistency and appearance* – mucoid, liquid or bloody.
3. *Colour* : Normal sputum is clear and colourless. A yellow colour indicates pus and epithelial cells as seen in pneumonic process. Rus coloured sputum is due to decomposition of haemoglobin and is seen in pneumococcal pneumonia, a pulmonary gangrene.
4. *Odour* Normal sputum is odourless.

Other abnormal constituents are :

1. Cheesy masses
2. Bronchial casts
3. Broncholitis (lung stones)
4. Dittrich's plugs
5. Foreign bodies
6. Parasites

Clinical Significance

The abnormal constituent of sputum is examined in common respiratory disorder.

Mycobacterial infection,
Mycotic (Fungal) disease,
Bronchial asthma,
Chronic bronchitis,
Lung abscess,
Pneumonia,
Pneumoconiosis,
Pulmonary embolism,
Heart disease, and
Viral infection.

SEMEN EXAMINATION

Semen analysis is carried out to evaluate infertility. Semen consists of spermatozoa suspended in seminal plasma. Spermatozoa comprises about 5% of the semen volume (derived from listis). The availability of semen renders possible direct examination of male germ cells, giving precious data that are not accessible for female germ cells. It includes the examination of :

(i) spermatozoa,
(ii) other cells present in semen,
(iii) Seminal fluid.

Normal sperm count range is from 60 to 150 million/ml with an average of 100 million/ml. Counts of less than 20 million/ml are considered distinctly abnormal. The presence of blood (*hematospermia*) is an indication of prostatis.

CEREBROSPINAL FLUID EXAMINATION

Cerebrospinal fluid is formed primarily in ventricular choroid plexuses by a combination of both, active process and ultracentrifugation.

It is examined to diagnose the suspected meningitis, subarachnoid haemorrhage, encephalitis, CNS syphilis and spinal cord tumor.

It is also examined to detect intracerebral haemorrhage (almost 80% of cases show blood or xanthochromia).

22

Chapter

Drug Interaction

The combination thereby or simultaneous use of two or more therapeutic agents has become a common practice to get better and prompt result. It is understood that hospitalized patients receive an average of 5-10 drugs and out-door patients may take 2-4 formulations.

Sometimes it is not safer to use these drugs in combination due to interaction problems. An interaction is said to occur when the effects of one drug is altered by the presence of another drug.

A drug interaction pair consists of object drug and the precipitant drug. The activity of the object drug is altered, the drug causing this change is the precipitant drug.

Occasionally, a drug may be an object drug in one interaction (e.g. phenytoin and cimetidine combination) and a precipitant drug in another interaction (e.g. doxycline and phenytoin combination). Rarely both interacting drugs are effected by each other (e.g. chloramphenicol and phenobarbitone combination).

Classification

Drug interactions are classified in the following ways :

1. **Consequences wise :** They are classified into two categories :
   (a) Beneficial,
   (b) Adverse drug interactions.

   Beneficial interactions are not frequently reported but in certain conditions they have been used to minimize the risk of a particular form of therapy or to improve its therapeutic efficacy, for example :

(i) Combination of sulphamethoxazole with trimethoprim is used to enhance the antibacterial effect of either therapeutic effect.

(ii) Combination of carbidopa with levodopa. Levodopa is the main drug, useful in parkinsonism. Carbidopa increases its effect by preventing its decarboxylation, consequently this makes more levodopa available for transport to brain so it reduces the dose of levodopa which decreases the toxicity.

(iii) Combination of different hypotensive drugs (e.g. β-receptor blocking drugs and diuretics) is used to get additive effects.

(iv) Combination of different antibiotics (e.g. ampicillin and cloxacilin) is in practice for better result.

(v) Various types of cytotoxic drugs are used in cancer therapy to increase therapeutic efficacy.

Adverse drug interaction results with drug that antagonize each other. Examples of this type of interaction include morphine and nalorphine (opposite physiological action), cholinestrase inhibitors and atropine (opposite physiological action).

2. **Sitewise :** On the basis of site, adverse reactions may be (a) external or (b) internal.

   (a) **External :** There are many physical and chemical incompatibilities when drugs are mixed in infusion, vials, syringes, etc. Precipitation or inactivation may occur.

   (b) **Internal :** In this adverse reaction is at body site or system (e.g. gastrointestinal tract, liver) or site of drug action (e.g. cell membrane, receptor site).

   For example atropine competitively blocks pilocarpine action at muscarinic receptors, coadministration of penicillins and tetracyclines (HCl) causes precipitation in intravenous fluid. Penicillins cause the inactivation of gentamicin if given together in intravenous fluid.

3. **Mechanism-wise** drug interactions can be classified on the basis of their mechanism as follows :

   A. **Pharmacokinetic drug interaction :** It occurs as a result of altered drug absorption, distribution, metabolism and exceration.

      1. **Altered drug absorption :** It may be due to following reasons :

         (i) **Physiochemical interaction :** Change in gastric pH

by one drug (for e.g. antacids-cimetidine, ranitidine) which affects the ionisation of another drug and so absorption of aspirin remains unionised at the stomach pH, so drug is rapidly absorbed from stomach but use of antacid with aspirin reduces the absorption due to alternation of pH.

Chelation of tetracycline in patients receiving iron/calcium preparation occurs, which results in poor absorption.

Activated charcoal absorbs many drugs in the stomach and so prevent their absorption.

(ii) **Altered gastrointestinal motility :** It affects the rates of drug absorption.

For example propantheline which delays gastric emptying and reduces intestinal motility will cause hinderance in absorption of many drugs, e.g., digoxin, quinidine. Similarly narcotic analgesics, e.g. morphine may delay the absorption.

Metclopropamide increases gastric emptying and intestinal motility and so causes rapid absorption of drug from the upper small intestine.

(iii) **Change in bacterial flora :** Intestinal flora may play important role in synthesizing vitamin K, essential for normal blood clotting or may reactive some inactive drug metal excreted via bile by deconjugating them. Antibiotics may interact with these drugs by modifying or eliminating intentinal flora.

(iv) **Changes in mucosal function :** Drug with specific gastrointestinal tract toxicity (e.g. colchicine) may damage the gastrointestinal mucosa or block active transport and so alter the absorption rate of the drug.

(v) **Blood flow :** The better the blood supply to an area where a drug being absorbed, the greater the concentration gradient and faster the absorption rate.

2. **Altered drug distribution :** Some drugs are highly bound to plasma proteins, for example coumarins, salphonylureas and phenytoin. Co-administration of a drug, which can displace the former from their binding sites, will cause an increased pharmacological activity and possibly toxicity. Trichloroacetic acid, a metabolite or chloral hydrate, may displace

warfarin from its binding sites (plasma protein) and so increases the anticoagulant activity which results in bleeding tendency.

Similarly, methotrexate, an anticancer drug, is displaced by some sulphonamides and a granulocytosis may result.

3. **Altered drug metabolism :**

   (i) **Inuction of hepatic microsomal enzymes :** Certain drugs, e.g. barbiturates, alcohol, phenylbutazone and some anticonvulsants, are potent inducers of hepatic microsomal enzymes. The simultaneous use of these drugs with any other drug, which is normally metabolized by this route, will result in increased metabolism or clearance of the latter with reduced therapeutic efficacy if the parent compound is the effect mediator but possibly increased if effect is due to a metabolite. For example, interaction of barbiturates with warfarin results in decreased anticoagulant effect. Interaction of tolbutamide with alcohol/phenytoin/rifampicillin results in decreased hypoglycemic effect.

   (ii) **Inhibition of hepatic microsomal enzymes :** Some drugs inhibit the activity of microsomal enzymes and so the metabolism of other drugs.

4. **Altered drug excretion :**

   (i) **Competition for active tubular secretion :** Active tubular secretion of many drug occurs in proximal limb of the loop of Henle. If two drugs, which are normally secreted in this way, are co-administered in large doses, competition may lead to an interaction whereby greater then expected amount of one or other are retained in the body. For example, interaction occurs between probenecid and pencillin in which probenecid is used to prolong the action of penicillin.

   (ii) **Change in urine pH :** Reabsorption of drugs is decreased in renal tubule by changing the pH of urine. It is most likely encouraged as, for example, in salicyiate or phenobarbitone poisoning where alkalinization of the urine will increase elimination of these drugs. Similarly acidifiers, e.g. ascorbic acid and ammonium chloride, are used to increase the elimination rate of amphetamine, fenfuramine and quinidine.

B. **Pharmacodynamic drug interaction :** It occurs as follows :

1. **Drugs having similar pharmacological effect :** A patient receiving hypnotic may develop an allergic skin reaction and for this, he receives an antihistamine which itself has central nervous system depressed effects. The combined effects may be sufficient to produce serious sedation which cannot be obtained from either of these drugs.
   Similar effects are observed with the use of hypnotics and alcohol (increased CNS depression), narcotic analgesics and tranquilizer (increased CNS depression), digoxin and quinidine (bradycardia), β-receptor stimulants and theophylline.
2. **Drugs having opposite pharmacological effects :** When a patient is receiving pilocarpine (cholinergic drug) for glaucoma (eye diseases) and at the same time for abdominal pain may be prescribed with an anticholinergic drug, then interocular pressure may be altered by the anticholinergic drug.
3. **Change in electrolytic and fluid balance :** Drugs, e.g. diuretics, that cause potassium depletion may potentiate the effects of digitalis and non-polarizing muscle relaxant but antagonize the effect of lignocaine, quinidine and procainamide.

DRUG-DRUG INTERACTIONS

Table 22.1. Analgesic drug interactions

Salicylates : All salicylates: aspirin, choline magnesium salicylate, choline salicylate, magnesium salicylate, sodium salicylate, sodium thiosalicylate

Interacting drug	*Possible effect*	*Clinical advise*
• Antacids (in large doses) or • Corticosteroids	Decreased salicylate effectiveness from hastened salicylate excretion	• Warm the patient against taking large doses of antacids To prevent possible GI distress, advise him to take aspirin with a glass of milk or with food • Assess the patient to determine the effectiveness of aspirin therapy
• Probenecid -do- • Sulfinpyrazone	Gout from increased serum uric acid levels, interaction blocks uric acid excretion	• Monitor serum uric acid levels • Assess the patient for signs and symptoms of gout, for example, joint pain and inflammation, especially in the toes. Teach the patient to recognize the report gout symptoms

		• Instruct the patient to avoid over-the-counter products containing aspirin. Also advise him to avoid alcohol and foods high in purine, such as coffee. These substances increase uric acid levels
• Carbonic anhydrase inhibitors, e.g. acetazolamide	Either salicylate toxicity or decreased salicylate effectiveness. Toxicity results from increased penetration of salicylic acid into central nervous system. Decreased effectiveness results from alkaline urine, which hastens salicylate excretion	• Watch for signs and symptoms of salicylate toxicity, such as hyperpnea, lethargy, vomiting, tinnitus, hearing loss, and dizziness • Check for lack of salicylate effectiveness

Table 22.2. Annticoagulant drug interactions

Warfarin and Dicumarol

Interacting drug	*Possible effect*	*Clinical advise*
• Alcohol	Bleeding from additive hypoprothrombinemic effect, or decreased anticoagulant effect from enhanced warfarin metabolism	• Monitor prothrombin time for deviations from the patient's baseline value • Monitor the patient's haemoglobin and hematocrit values. A decrease in these values may indicate bleeding • Watch for bleeding and signs of occult bleeding, e.g. melena, cloudy urine, or coffee-ground vomitus • Instruct him to avoid alcoholic beverages in excess Over-the-counter products containing alcohol, such as liquid cough and cold preparations, can be used with caution
• Salicylates	Bleeding from displacement of warfarin from protein-binding sites and from additive hypoprothrombinemic effect	• Monitor prothrombin time • Monitor the patient's haemoglobin and hematocrit values. A decrease in these values may indicate bleeding • Watch for bleeding and signs of occult bleeding, e.g. melena, cloudy urine or coffe-ground vomitus

(Contd.)

Interacting drug	*Possible effect*	*Clinical advise*
		• Instruct the patient to avoid aspirin and over-the-counter products containing aspirin • Tell him to report excessive or unexplained bleeding or bruising to his doctor
• Carbamazepine -do- • Barbiturates -do- • Glutethimide or • Rifampin	Decreased anticoagulant effect from enhanced warfarin or dicumarol metabolism	• Monitor prothrombin time • Watch for signs of increased clotting effect • Adjust anticoagulant dosage, as ordered
• Phenylbutazone or • Oxyphenbutazone or • Chloral hydrate	Bleeding from displacement of warfarin or dicumarol from protein binding sites	• Use extreme caution when giving any of these drugs with an oral anticoagulant • Monitor prothrombin time • Monitor the patient's hemoglobin and hematocrit values. A decrease in these values may indicate bleeding • Watch for bleeding and signs of bleeding, e.g. melena, cloudy urine or coffe-ground vomitus • Notify the doctor if the patient develops GI distress or other signs that might indicate bleeding
• Quinidine	Bleeding from additive hypoprothrombinemic effect	• Use these drugs together with caution • Monitor prothrombin tim • Monitor the patient's haemoglobin hematocrit values. A decrease in these values may indicate bleeding • Watch for bleeding and signs of bleeding, e.g. melena, cloudy urine or coffee-ground vomitus
• Clofibrate or • Disulfiram or • Thyroid hormones	Bleeding, mechanism unknown	• Monitor prothrombin time • Monitor the patient's haemoglobin and hematocri values. A decrease in these values may indicate bleeding • Watch for bleeding and signs of bleeding, e.g. melena, cloudy urine or coffee-ground vomitus
• Cholestyramine • Colestipol	Decreased anticoagulant effect from decreased absorption	• Monitor prothrombin time • Administer the drugs approximately 6 hours apart, if possible, to minimize the interaction

Table 22.3. Oral antidiabetic drug interactions

All orally administered antidiabetics e.g. chlorpropamide and tolbutamide

Interacting drug	*Possible effect*	*Clinical advise*
• Alcohol	Antabuse-like reaction from acetaldehyde accumulation, also possible hypoglycemia from additive effect	• Instruct the patient to avoid alcohol and over-the-counter products containing alcohol (e.g., liquid cough and cold preparations) • Teach him to recognize the symptoms of an antabuse-like reaction: sweating, diarrhea, nausea and vomiting and headache
• Beta blockers, e.g. propranolol, nadolol, pindolol and timolol	Hypoglycemia without the usual signs and symptoms. Beat blockers inhibit hypoglycemic signs and symptoms mediated by the adrenergic nervous system and may block rebound glycogenolysis	• Monitor serum glucose levels regularly • Instruct the patient to adhere to his prescribed diet • To minimize this interaction, the doctor may order a cardioselective beta blocker, such as atenolol or metaprolol
• Chloramphenicol	Hypoglycemia from blocked metabolism of antidiabetic drugs	• Monitor serum glucose levels regularly • Check the patient for signs and symptoms of hypoglycemia, sweating, confusion, pallor and hunger
• Oxyphenbutazone -do- • Phenylbutazone	Hypoglycemia from displacement of antidiabetic from protein-binding sites and possibly from inhibited excretion	• Avoid these combinations, if possible • Closely monitor serum glucose levels • Observe the patient for signs and symptoms of hyperglycemia, anorexia, nausea and vomiting, lethargy thirst and polyuria • Tell him to avoid over-the-counter products containing sugar
• Rifampicin	Hyperglycemia and poor control of diabetes from increased metabolism of antidiabetic drug	• Monitor serum glucose levels • Test urine for glucose and acetone regularly • Check the patient for signs and symptoms of hyperglycemia, anorexia, nausea and vomiting, lethargy thirst and polyuria • Tell him to avoid over-the-counter products containing sugar

(Contd.)

Interacting drug	*Possible effect*	*Clinical advise*
• Sulfomamides	Hypoglycemia, mainly from displacement of antidiabetic drug form protein-binding sites	• Monitor serum glucose levels • Observe the patient for signs and symptoms of hypoglycemia, seating, confusion, pallor and hunger
• Fenfluramine	Hypoglycemia from additive effect	• Monitor serum glucose levels • Observe the patient for signs and symptoms of hypoglycemia, seating, confusion, pallor and hunger
• MAO inhibitors or • Salicylates (in high doses)	Hypoglycemia, mechanism unknown	• Monitor serum glucose levels • Observe the patient for signs and symptoms of hypoglycemia, sweating, confusion, pallor and hunger
• Dicumarol	Hypoglycemia or bleeding form displacement of either drug from protein-binding produced	• Monitor serum glucose levels and prothrombin time
• Thiazide diuretics	Thiazide-produced hypoglycemia, which antagonizes antidiabetic action	• Monitor serum glucose levels • Test urine for glucose and acetone regularly • Observe the patient for signs and symptoms of hypoglycemia, anorexia, nausea and vomiting lethargy thirst and polyuria

CARDIOVASCULAR DRUGS INTERACTION

Table 22.4. Antiarrhythmic drug interactions

Lidocaine

Interacting drug	*Possible effect*	*Clinical advise*
• Disopyramide or • Phenytoin	Myocardial depression, congestive heart failure and dysrhythmias from additive effect	• Observe the patient for signs and symptoms of myocardial depression (such as hypotension and bradycardia), congestive heart failure and dysrhythmias • Obtain regular EKG readings, as ordered
• Beta adrenergic blockers or • Cimetidine	Lidocaine toxicity from inhibited lidocaine metabolism	• Observe the patient for signs and symptoms of lidocaine toxicity, such as sedation, confusion and seizures • Also check for signs and symptoms of myocardial depression (such as hypotension and bradycardia), congestive heart failure and dysrhythmias

		• Monitor plasma lidocaine levels
• Neuromuscular blocking agents, for example, succinyl-choline	Increased neuromuscular blocking effect, causing prolonged respiratory depression, mechanism unknown	• Provide mechanical respiratory support, as required • Closely monitor the patient for respiratory depression and apnea

Quinidine

Interacting drug	*Possible effect*	*Clinical advise*
• Drugs that alter urine pH, e.g., vitamin C and carbonic anhydrase inhibitors, such as acetazolamide and antacids	Quinine toxicity, causing myocardial depression and dysrhythmias, form urine alkalinization that increases quinidine reabsorption, or decreased quinidine effectiveness from urine acidification that decreases reabsorption	• Monitor urine pH and plasma quinidine levels. Therapeutic plasma levels range from 1 to 6 mg/ml • Regularly check the patient's pulse and blood pressure • Monitor check the patient's pulse and blood pressure • Monitor his EKG readings for widening QRS complex and dysrhythmias • Teach the patient how to rest his urine pH at home
• Cimetidine	Quinidine toxicity from inhibited quinidine metabolism	• Monitor plasma quinidine levels. Therapeutic levels range from 1 to 6 µg/ml • Regularly check the patient's pulse and blood pressure • Monitor his EKG readings for widening QRS complex and dysrhythmias • Adjust quinidine dosage, if ordered
• Barbiturates or • Phenytoin or • Rifampin	Decreased quinidine effect from increased quinidine metabolism	• Monitor plasma quinidine levels. Therapeutic levels range form 1 to 6 µg/ml • Regularly check the patient's pulse and blood pressure • Monitor his EKG readings for widening QRS complex and dysrhythmias • Assess the effectiveness of quinidine therapy
• Neuromuscular blocking agents, e.g., succinyl-choline	Increased neuromuscular blocking effect, causing prolonged respiratory depression, mechanism unknown	• Provide mechanical respiratory support, as required • Closely monitor the patient for respiratory depression and apnea • Regularly check the patient's pulse and blood pressure • Monitor his EKG reading for widening QRS complex and dysrhythmias

Table 22.5. Antihypertensive drug interactions

All antihypertensive causing orthostatic hypotension e.g., sympatholytic drugs

Interacting drug	*Possible effect*	*Clinical advise*
• Phenothiazines, e.g., chlorpromazine and prochlorperazine or • Nitrates, e.g. nitroglycerin and iso-sorbide dinitrate	Orthostatic hypotension from additive hypotensive effect	• Monitor the patient for orthostatic changes in blood pressure and pulse while he's lying, sitting and standing • Advise the patient to stand slowly to avoid dizziness • Administer nitrates while the patient is lying down to avoid severe headache and symptomatic hypotension

Captopril

Interacting drug	*Possible effect*	*Clinical advise*
• Potassium or potassium-sparing diuretics (spironolactone, trimaterene and amiloride	Hyperkalemia from potassium retention caused by captopril	• Regularly monitor serum potassium and other electrolyte levels • Monitor EKG readings for widening of QRS complexes, tall T waves, and ventricular fibrillation • Check for other signs and symptoms of hyperkalemia, irritability, nausea and diarrhea
• Nonsteroidal anti-inflammatory agents, e.g. indomethacin and ibuprofen	Reduced antihypertensive effect from inhibition of endogenous prostaglandin synthesis	• Monitor the patient's blood pressure carefully for worsening hypertension. In this occurs, the doctor may discontinue the anti-inflammatory agent

Clonidine

Interacting drug	*Possible effect*	*Clinical advise*
• Levodopa	Reduced antiparkinsonian effectiveness from negation of levodopa activity	• Check for signs and symptoms of parkinsonism, facial grimacing, jerky arm and leg movements and bobbing head • As ordered, gradually discontinue clonidine over 24 hours and replace with another antihypertensive drug
• Tricyclic antidepressants	Decreased antihypertensive effectiveness, mechanism unknown	• Monitor the patient's blood pressure carefully • Emphasize the importance of having his blood pressure checked regularly after he leaves the hospital • Adjust the clonidine dosage as ordered

Guanethidine

Interacting drug	*Possible effect*	*Clinical advise*
• Tricyclic antidepressants or • Amphetamines and amphetamine-like drugs, e.g., fenfluramine or • Phenothiazines or • Haloperidol	Decreased antihypertensive effectiveness form inhibition of guanethidine's neuronal uptake	• Avoid these drug combinations, if possible • If the doctor orders such a combination, suggest that he increase the quanethidine dosage • Monitor the patient's blood pressure carefully • emphasize the importance of having his blood pressure checked regularly after he leaves the hospital
• Sympathomimetics, e.g. dopamine, ephedrine, phenylephrine, and norepinephrine	Severe hypertension from drug antagonism that reduces guanethidine's effectiveness, and increased sympathetic stimulation	• Avoid this drug combination • Warm the patient taking guanethidine to avoid over-the-counter products containing sympathomimetics • Advise him to consult the pharmacist before using any over-the-counter product

Interacting drug	*Possible effect*	*Clinical advise*
Prazosin		
• Beta adrenergic blockers	Acute hypotension from synergistic increase in prazosin effects	• Monitor the patient carefully for acute hypotension, especially following the first prazosin dose. first dose should be given at bedtime • Emphasize the importance of having his blood pressure checked regularly after he leaves the hospital

Table 22.6. β-Adrenergic blocker interactions

All beta adrenergic blockers : atenolol, metaprolol, nadolol, pindolol, propranolol, timolol

Interacting drug	*Possible effect*	*Clinical advise*
• All bronchodilators, e.g. albuterol, aminophylline, metaproterenol, terbutaline	Bronchospasm and wheezing from antagonistic action of beta blocker	• Check the patient's history for asthma • Monitor him for signs and symptoms or pulmonary disorders, wheezing, shortness of breath, restlessness, increased pulse rate, and dizziness

(Contd.)

Interacting drug	*Possible effect*	*Clinical advise*
		• Instruct the patient to report breathing problems and warn him not to stop taking the drug without consulting the doctor • To minimize this interaction, the doctor may order cardioselective beta blocker, such as atenolol or metoprolol
• Theophylline	Reduced theophylline effectiveness from antagonistic action of beta blocker	• Monitor the patient for theophylline effectiveness • Monitor plasma theophylline levels. Therapeutic levels range from 10 to 20 μg/ml. If necessary, suggest that the doctor increase the theophylline dosage • Assess the patient for breathing problems. Instruct him to report breathing problems. • To minimize this interaction, the doctor may be order a cardio-selective beta blockers, such as atenolol or metoprolol

Metoprolol and Propranolol

Interacting drug	*Possible effect*	*Clinical advise*
• Chlorpromazine	Increased beta blockers effect form antagonistic action of beat blocker	• Monitor the patient's blood pressure and pulse rate • If necessary, suggest that the doctor decrease the beta blocker dosage
• Barbiturates	Decreased beta blocker effectiveness form increase first-pass metabolism of barbiturates	• Monitor the patient's blood pressure and pulse rate • If necessary, suggest that the doctor increase the beat blocker dosage

Propranolol only

Interacting drug	*Possible effect*	*Clinical advise*
• Cimetidine	Beta blocker toxicity form inhibited metabolism or decreased first-pass effect	• Monitor the patient's blood pressure and pulse rate • If necessary, suggest that the doctor decreased the propranolol dosage

Table 22.7. Calcium channel blocker interactions

All calcium blockers : diltiazem, nifedipine, verapamil

Interacting drug	*Possible effect*	*Clinical advise*
• Beta blockers	Heart block form negative inotropic effect of both agents. *Note* : This interaction is somewhat more significant with verapamil	• Observe the patient for signs and symptoms of congestive heart failure, such as shortness of breath and swollen ankles. Teach him to recognize and report these signs and symptoms • Check for breathing problems and light-headedness • Instruct the patient to count his pulse rate and to report an abnormally slow rate (less than 50 beats/minute or as specified by the doctor) • Tell him to take the drugs only in the prescribed dosages and to consult a doctor before discounting the drug, taking additional medications, or drinking alcoholic beverages
• Disopyramide	Heart block form inhibition of AV conduction by both drugs. *Note* : This interaction is somewhat more significant with verapamil	• Follow the same guidelines listed above
• Antihypertensives	Additive hypotension. *Note* : This interaction is somewhat more significant with nifedipine	• Periodically check blood pressure and pulse while the patient is lying down, sitting and standing • Advise him to sit and stand slowly to avoid dizziness
• Digoxin	Digitalis toxicity form increased plasma digoxin levels. *Note* : This interaction is somewhat more significant with verapramil	• Observe the patient for signs and symptoms of digitalis toxicity, nausea and vomiting, anorexia, diarrhea, dyshythmias and green- or yellow-tinted vision • Monitor plasma digoxin levels. Therapeutic levels range from 0.7 to 2.0 ng/ml • If necessary, suggest that the doctor reduce the digoxin dosage

Table 22.8. Cardiactonic drug interactions

All digitalis glycosides, e.g., digitalis, digitoxin, digoxin

Interacting drug	*Possible effect*	*Clinical advise*
• Potassium-wasting diuretics, e.g. thiazide diuretics and loop diuretics	Digitalis toxicity from hypokalemia	• Monitor serum potassium levels • Check EKG readings for ST segment depression • Observe the patient for signs and symptoms of digitalis toxicity, nausea and vomiting, anorexia, diarrhea, dysrhythmias, and green- or yellow-tinted vision
• Thyroid hormones is very high doses	Reduced effectiveness of digitalis glycoside, mechanism unknown	• Monitor the patient for decreased response todigitalis glycoside. *Note*: A patient with a hyperthyroid condition may experience the same interaction

Digitoxin only

Interacting drug	*Possible effect*	*Clinical advise*
• Cholestyramine or • Colestipol	Decreased digitoxin effect form digitoxin binding to cholestyramine or colestipol in the GI tract	• If possible, avoid this combination • If the patient must receive this combination, increase the digitoxin dosage as ordered and monitor plasma digotoxin levels • Therapeutic levels range from 15 to 30 ng/ml

Digoxin only

Interacting drug	*Possible effect*	*Clinical advise*
• Anticholinergics	Digoxin toxicity from increased intestinal absorption of digoxin	• Check the patient for signs and symptoms of digoxin toxicity, nausea and vomiting, anorexia, diarrhea, dysrhythmias and green- or yellow-tinted vision
• Metoclopramide	Decreased digoxin effect from decreased intestinal absorption of digoxin tablets	• Substitute digoxin tablets with digoxin elixir or liquid-filled capsules (Lanoxicaps), as ordered
• Quinidine	Digoxin toxicity form altered digoxin distribution	• Monitor plasma digoxin levels. Therapeutic levels range from 0.7 to 2 ng/ml • Reduce the digoxin dosage, as ordered • Check the patient for signs and symptoms of digoxin toxicity, nausea and vomiting, anorexia, diarrhea, dysrhythmias and green- or yellow-tinted vision

Table 22.9. Diuretics drug interactions

All potassium-wasting diuretics, e.g. thiazide diuretics and loop diuretics

Interacting drug	*Possible effect*	*Clinical advise*
• Corticosteroids	Hypokalemia from additive effect	• Monitor serum potassium levels • Check the patient for signs and symptoms of hypokalemia, muscle cramps, irregular heart rate and ST segment depression on EKG

All potassium-sparing diuretics : amiloride, spironolactone, triamterene

Interacting drug	*Possible effect*	*Clinical advise*
• Potassium supplements	Hyperkalemia from potassium retention	• Monitor serum potassium levels • Check EKG readings for widening of QRS complexes, tall T waves and ventricular fibrillation • Observe the patient for other signs and symptoms of hyperkalemia, muscular weakness, paralysis and abdominal cramps • Instruct the patient no minimize intake of food high in potassium (such as fruits and leafy green vegetables) and to avoid drastic dietary changes

Spironolactone only

Interacting drug	*Possible effect*	*Clinical advise*
• Aspirin	Reduced diuretic effect from negation of renal action of spirolactone	• Tell the patient to avoid over-the-counter products containing aspirin

Table 22.10. Gastro-intestinal drug interaction

All Antacids

Interacting drug	*Possible effect*	*Clinical advise*
• All enteric-coated products, including some forms of aspirin, e.g. Ecosprin	Premature drug dissolution in the stomach, antacids destroy enteric coating	• Administer 1 hour apart

Antacids containing calcium, magnesium or aluminium

Interacting drug	*Possible effect*	*Clinical advise*
• Iron salts	Decreased iron absorption from iron precipitation, causing decreased response in treating anemia	• Administer drugs 2 hours apart • Monitor the patient for decreased hematologic response to iron salt therapy

Cimetidine

Interacting drug	*Possible effect*	*Clinical advise*
• All benzodiazepines (except lorazepam, oxazepam and temazepam)	Excessive sedation form decreased metabolism of benzodiazepines	• Decrease benzodiazepine dosage as ordered • Check the patient for unusual fatigue • Instruct the patient to take the drug exactly as prescribed and to notify the doctor before adding other medications, alcoholic beverages, or over-the-counter product containing alcohol • Tell him to notify the doctor if he experiences slurred speech, unsteady gait or extreme fatigue
• Theophylline	Theophylline toxicity from decreased theophylline metabolism	• Monitor plasma theophylline levels. Therapeutic levels range from 10 to 20 μg/ml • Check the patient for signs and symptoms of theophylline toxicity: anorexia, nausea and vomiting, headache, tachycardia, dizziness and restlessness

Table 22.11. Vitamins interactions

Vitamin B_6

Interacting drug	*Possible effect*	*Clinical advise*
• Levodopa	Decreased antiparkinson effectiveness of levodopa from increased levodopa metabolism	• Avoid administering vitamin B_6 to a patient who's receiving levodopa, or ask the doctor to substitute levodopa with levodopa-carbidopa (Sinemet) to avoid this interaction

Folic acid

Interacting drug	*Possible effect*	*Clinical advise*
• Sulfassalazine	Reduced folic acid effectiveness form decreased GI absorption of folic acid	• If folic acid replacement is required, make sure the doctor orders a parenteral route

Vitamin B_{12}

Interacting drug	*Possible effect*	*Clinical advise*
• Para-aminosalicylic acid	Reduced vitamin B_{12} effectiveness form decreased GI absorption of vitamin B_{12}	• Administer vitamin B_{12} by a parenteral route, as ordered
• Chloramphenicol	Decreased effectiveness of vitamin B_{12} in treatment of anemia from chloramphenicol-induced inhibition of haemoglobin syntheses	• Be aware that the patient's response to vitamin B_{12} therapy may be delayed • Monitor the patient's complete blood cell count, as ordered

Drug Food Interaction

Food alters drug therapy in the following way :

(i) Alteration of absorption,
(ii) Alteration of distribution,
(iii) Alteration of biotransformation, and
(iv) Alteration of excretion.

Factors that Affect Food and Drug Interaction

The overall interaction of food and drug will vary considerably with the kinds and types of food or beverages, the amount of food material retained and absorbed along the gastrointestinal tract the time of day or night the food was ingested, the presence or absence of active ingredients and time-release formulations, and the presence or absence of physiological factors that alter a drug's absorption, distribution, metabolism and excretion.

Surface Area

When there is a reduced exposure to surface area in the stomach due to the presence of food, there is reduction in the actual amount of the drug absorbed by the body. The absorption of antibiotics has been found to be impaired when taken with foods. Low levels of the antibiotics were noted in the blood and in urinary excretions. Furosemide is another drug in which absorption is impaired by food substances. A delay or diminished urinary output was noted when furosemide was given with breakfast. Drugs that interact with ingested foods are more likely to be dissolved by acids or absorbed by proteins. The drug is then eliminated through the fecal contents. Moreover, if the drug is administered in low doses, the above interactions are more likely to occur, with consequently reduced therapeutic effects. Studies have shown that factors such as a large surface area and a high concentration of the drug to promote a more rapid dissolution process. Usually, when drugs are more rapidly dissolved they are more completely absorbed by the body.

In contrast certain antimicrobial agents have especially slow and poor absorption rates when given on an empty stomach. These drugs have been found to have high absorption rates when they are administered with fatty foods at mealtime. Griseofulvin is more completely absorbed when administered on an empty stomach or with a high-fat breakfast than when administered with a high-fat dinner. These drugs are not affected therapeutically when administered with a high-protein or high-carbohydrate diet.

Temperature

The temperature of the environment is yet another physical factor affecting drug dissolution and absorption. When drugs are ingested with a hot food or beverage, there is usually a faster rate of dissolution. Cold products have the opposite effect, a slower rate of dissolution takes place when cold foods or beverages are consumed.

Coated Tablets

Simple coated tablets are covered with sugar or a water-soluble material to cover up drugs with objectionable tastes or odours. Because coated tablets are designed to control the release rates of their ingredients, a longer disintegration period is expected. Enteric coating helps resist dissolution in gastric fluid but allows disintegration in intestine. These are used for drugs that are inactivated by the stomach or irritate the stomach, mucosa. Interference with "timed-release" tables occurs when administered with hot foods or beverages. The drug dissolves more readily when it is in contact with hot products, causing a release of all of the drug's ingredients within a very short period of time.

In addition, dairy products or antacids can cause an untimely release of coated tablets. When bisacodyl is dissolved by dairy products in the stomach, gastric irritation and bleeding can result. Therefore, all coated tablets need to be given on an empty stomach with a full glass (8 oz) of water.

Dietary Metals

Foods containing dietary metals such as calcium, magnesium and iron may also be influencing variables on a drug's dissolution and absorption processes. Tetracycline, demeclocycline, chlorotetracycline and doxycycline are only a few antibiotics found to bind in varying degrees with metals. Consequently, these drugs will not be dissolved or absorbed by the body. Antibiotics are often given with meals because of convenience. This, as well as the administration of these drugs with the all-too-common milk product, reduce the therapeutic effect of these drugs. It is extremely important to emphasize to the client not to use foods or beverages, especially dairy products, that are high in metals (magnesium, calcium and iron) in conjunction with the drug therapy.

Foodstuffs that are high in phosphates and phytates, such as cereals, brown breads and milk products, can significantly lower the absorption of zinc and calcium. Coffee also has a similar effect that is due to the poor solubility and absorption characteristics of zinc sulfate. Because zinc sulfate is highly irritating to the gastrointestinal tract, it is important to advice individuals to consume foods and beverages other than coffee, cereal, brown bread, and milk.

Individuals taking iron supplements need to be aware of the need for vitamin C for iron absorption. Vitamin C in citrus fruits provides an acidic environment in the small intestine that is needed for the iron supplement to be absorbed by the body. Milk products and antacids, however, increase the quantity of insoluble salts in the body, which interferes with the absorption of iron. This has greater implications for pregnant women who need metals from dairy products and ulcer patients who need the protective coating of antacids as well as supplemental iron.

Other Dietary Compounds

Antipyretic and analgesic agents (such as acetaminophen) have shown variations of peak levels in the blood that are related to the content of dietary components. Meals high in carbohydrates significantly impair acetaminophen absorption. Therefore, crackers, breads and cereals should not be given within 2 hours before or after acetaminophen is administered.

Foods containing high quantities of active amines (aged cheese, chocolate, beer, yeast, Chianti wines, salmani and sausage) have the potential to trigger a hypertensive crisis in those individuals on monoamine oxidase (MAO) inhibitors. The MAO inhibitors potentiate the vasoconstriction effects of these amines, which can lead to dangerously high levels of hypertension. Consequently, sudden severe headaches, intracranial hemorrhage, and death can occur. MAO inhibitors include pargyline and procarbazine, which can also protentiate and intensify the actions of many other drugs.

Diets that influence the urine pH in the body also affect the elimination and activity of drugs normally excreted in the urine. Foods that increase the acidic level in the urine, namely bacon, cakes, cheese, eggs, meats and fish will potentiate the activity of weakly acidic drugs. Coumarin, acetylsalicylic acid, sulfonamides and barbiturates are few examples of acidic drugs reabsorbed by the kidney's tubular system. Food products such as milk, almonds, vegetables, and fruits increase the alkaline level of the urine pH and thus influence the weakly basic drug's pharmacologic activities. Morphine, meperidine, quinine, reserpine, aminophylline, and antihistamines are only a short list of drugs that may undergo tubular reabsorption, thereby potentiating the drug's activities.

23

Chapter

Adverse Drug Reactions

Adverse drug reactions are defined as any undesired or unintended effect of drug treatment. This is a broad definition and has mix validity for patients as it also includes excessive pharmacological effects as adverse drug reactions. For example, antidiabetic drugs is beneficial in diabetes mellitus but sometimes hypoglycemia is developed due to excessive pharmacological effect and so regarded as adverse drug effect.

Classification of Adverse Drug Reactions

Adverse drug reactions are due to following reasons, accordingly they are classified :

1. Excessive therapeutic effects
2. Secondary pharmacological effects
3. Idiosyncrasy
4. Allergic reactions
5. Genetic make up of the patients
6. Sudden drug withdrawal
7. Drug interactions

Each of these different reasons causes adverse drug reactions which are influenced by other factors like recommended dosage, formulation, route of administration and patient factors such as age, sex, weight, presence of underlying disease of kidney or liver disease.

1. Excessive Pharmacological Effect

Excessive pharmacological activity generally appears due to over dosage of a drug. This is particularly troublesome with cardioactive, hypotensive, hypoglycemia and central nervous system depressive agents, For example, hypotensive agent used in hypertension, in excess dose causes profound hypotension.

Adverse reaction due to excess pharmacological effects may also appear at usual therapeutic dose in certain conditions. These include :

(i) Patients with kidney disease particularly those who have lost more than 70% kidney function.

(ii) Hypoaalbuminemia which may be due to failure of albumin production as in liver disease or albumin loss as in nephrotic syndrome.

(iii) Patients at the extremes of the age range, i.e. infants and neonates.

Adverse reaction in these conditions can be minimized by dose adjustment after knowing the pharmacokinetic behaviour of an administered drug.

2. Secondary Pharmacological Effects

Drugs have several pharmacological actions at usual therapeutic dose but it is prescribed solely for one of these beneficial actions. For example, antihistamines are prescribed for their antiallergic skin reactions or for their antinausea effects, but they also produce drowsiness du to central nervous system depression (secondary pharmacological effects). This action may be of little importance for patients lying on bed but it may have disastrous consequences if a patient is motor driver. This effect may be greatly exacerbated if the patient is also taking hypnotics, tranquilizer, cough suppressant as medicines or is consuming alcohol.

3. Idiosyncrasy

The term, idiosyncrasy is used for unusual, unexpected drug effect which cannot be readily explained or predicted. It also includes drug induced foetal abnormalities such as phocomelia developing in offspring of mother exposed to thalidomide. Thalidomide develops as potential terogenecity if given to mothers during initial period of gestation when the limb buds are formed. Structural changes at molecular level occur in the foetal skeletal and neurological tissue but the nature of these changes are known for the development of foetal abnormalities-phocomelia.

Drug induced cancer is a idiosyncratic reaction. For example :

(i) Vaginal adenocarcinoma in girls with prolonged use of stilbosterol.

(ii) Tumors in kidney pelvis with prolonged use of stilbosterol.

(iii) Uterine cancer in patients with prolonged use of oestrogens.

(iv) Lymphnoid tumors in patients receiving long term immunosuppressive therapy with azathioprine, cyclophosphamide and other similar agent.

4. Allergic Drug Reactions

Allergic drug reactions range from very mild reactions to anaphylaxis and death may occur rarely after exposure to wide variety of drugs.

Characteristics of allergic adverse reactions are as follows :

(i) The reaction do not resemble to the expected pharmacological effect of the drug.

(ii) There is delay between the first exposure to the drug and development of the allergic reaction.

(iii) Allergic reaction re-occurs on repeated exposure even to traces of allergenic drugs.

Mechanism of allergic drug reaction can be explained on immunological basis. Drug or its metabolite combines with circulating plasma protein to form antigen. When an individual comes in contact with such antigen, antibody formation (resensitized or allergic response) takes place. Such individual when re-exposed to the same drug, antigen reacts with the antibodies and liberates the mediators of allergic reaction from mast cells, e.g. kinins, histamine, serotonins and prostaglandins. Symptoms of an allergic reaction become apparent which are characteristic of the mediator and not the drug. Some example of allergic reactions and their initiating drugs are shown in Table 23.1.

Table 23.1. Allergic drug reaction

Allergic response	*Allergic drug reaction*
Anaphylaxis	Penicillins
Haemolytic anaemia (Red blood cell destruction)	Penicillin, sulphonamide, guinidine
Leucopenia (White blood cell destruction)	Sulphonamides, phenylbutazone
Skin rashes	Sulpha drugs, penicillin, barbituriates
Hepatitis	Phenothiazine, methyl dopa
Nephritis	Methicillin, oxacillin, rifampicillin
Vasculitis	Sulpha drugs
Lupus syndrome	Procainamide, hydrazine, isoniazid

5. Genetically Determined Toxicity

Patients of selected selected genetic make up are at substantially greater then average risk for some specific drug toxicities. For example, glucose-6-phosphate dehydrogenase is involved in degradation of glucose for producing energy. Certain population in Africa and South East Asia are deficient in glucose-6-phosphate dehydrogenase and, therefore, there are substantial risks of developing haemolytic disease after the use of antimalarial drug-primaquine, sulphonamides, guinidine and nitrofurantoin.

Similarly there are other genetically determined toxicity. These include :

(i) Patients with porphyria are susceptible to CNS depressive agents like barbiturates.

(ii) Individual with pseudocholinestrase deficiency is highly susceptible to succinylcholine. They may develop paralysis and often apnoea.

(iii) Many drugs are detoxified in liver by acetylation. The ability of acetylation of many drugs in liver is variable between individuals. Slow acetylators have greater risk of toxicity for some drugs like isoniazide, procainamide, hydrallazine, phenelzine and dapsone.

6. Toxicity Following Drug Withdrawal

Tolerance occurs after prolong use of variety of drugs of narcotic analgesics, hypnotics, ethyl alcohol, some hypotensive agents (clonidine) and corticosteroid drugs. Sudden withdrawal of such drugs shows severe adverse effects.

In patients habituated to central nervous depressants such as ethyl alcohol, barbiturates and some benzodiazepines, withdrawal of the usual dose may produce marked agitation, tachycardia, confusion, delirium and convulsions.

Clonidine is used in hypertension but its sudden withdrawal may cause severe hypertension.

Long term of corticosteroid therapy is less common because it may cause atrophy of recipient's adrenal glands. Therefore, sudden withdrawal can precipitate an acute adrenal crisis (Addison's disease) in which the patients become profoundly weak, hypotensive and are collapsed. Such circumstances can be avoided by gradual removal of the corticosteroid over a period of weeks depending upon length of time they have been consumed.

7. Drug Interaction

Now-a-days many drugs are used in combination to get prompt relief. Sometimes these may interact together and cause adverse reactions (Chapter 21).

Adverse Reactions to Drugs

Adverse reactions to drugs take varying lengths of time to develop. Some become apparent immediately while others may require weeks or months to develop. Their severity may range from mild to catastrophic. Any body tissue or organ can be affected. Table 23.2 details the diseases due to some adverse drug reactions.

Table 23.2. Drug-induced diseases

Condition	*Examples of drug involved*
Joint pain	Rubella vaccine, sulfisoxazole penicillin, tetracycline, methylphenindate diazepam
Skin problems	
Dermatoses Acne Photosensitivity	Penicillins, bromides, thiazides corticosteroids, androgens, hydroxyzine, tetracycline, chloroquine, hydroxychloroquine, tolbutamide, chlorpropamide, vinblastine, anticonvulsants (phenytoin and trimethadione), barbiturates, phenothiazines, amitryptyline, 5-fluorouracil, quinidine, hydrochlorothiazide (topical), salicylates (topical), tretinoin (tropical), hexachlorophene
Gastrointestinal irritation and/or breeding	Anti-inflammatories such as aspirin and indomethacin, corticosteroids, antineoplastics
Cardiac arrest	Antiarrhythmics such as quinidine
Hepatotoxicity	Acetaminophen, alcohol, chloroform
Starch peritonitis	Starch applied to surgical gloves before sterilization and inadequately removed before surgery
Nephrotoxicity	Sulfonamides, uricosurics
Ototoxicity	Quinine, aspirin, streptomycin
Impaired sight	Oxygen (in new borns), corticosteroid
Thrombi	Oral contraceptives
Hypoglycemia	Insulin, oral hypoglycemics

(Cont

Condition	*Examples of drug involved*
Gangrene of an extremity	Propranolol, ergotamine
Changes in brain function	
Oversedation	Narcotic, analgesics, antihistamines, alcohol, phenylbutazone
Overstimulation	Decongestants, vasopressors
Psychosis	Corticosteroids, thyroid extract, amphetamines, alcohol, phenylbutazone
Bone marrow suppression	Chloramphenicol, phenylbutazone, ethosuximide, antineoplastics
Superinfection	Broad-spectrum antibiotics
Fluid and electrolyte imbalances	Diuretics, hormones such as estrogen and corticosteroids
Anaphylaxis	Penicillins
Teratogenetic birth defects	Thalidomide, alcohol, vitamin A, aspirin, metabisulfate (a preservative)
Acute allergic reactions	Cholinergics, penicillins
Cushing's syndrome	Corticosteroids
Drug dependence	
Addiction, habituation	Narcotic analgesics, tranquillizers
Deficiency due to organ atrophy	Corticosteroids
Benzyl alcohol poisoning (in infants)	Bacteriostatic NaCl solutions containing benzyl alcohol

Clients receiving relatively new drugs are particularly vulnerable to unexpected complications. The newer the drugs the greater the risk of unknown danger. However, adverse reactions to drug that have been well tolerated for extended periods of time can occur owing to changes in the ability of the client to metabolize or excrete the drug or because of inter-current illness. The identification of common reactions to a specific drug often requires 10 to 20 years of experience in therapeutic use. Even then some problems may not be recognized as being drug related. For example, aspirin was widely used for decades before its detrimental effects were acknowledged. The importance of careful observation and complete documentation of client response to medication cannot be overemphasized.

Side effects are those actions of a drug that are specifically desired in a treatment situation. No drug exert a single effect on the body;

rather, a spectrum of multiple effects occurs. A substance administered in one instance for a particular purpose may be used in another for a different effect. Which of the actions are termed therapeutic and which are deemed side effects depends upon the situation. Side effects are not all detrimental; many drugs are chosen for prescription in order to exploit their desirable side effects. For example, diazepam (Valium) is both a tranquilizer and a skeletal muscle relaxant. When administered to reduce anxiety, its relaxant properties are considered side effects. When used to treat low-back pain, tranquillization is considered a side effect. In the latter instance, the side effect is usually considered helpful, because the client often has difficulty adjusting to the immobility and pain associated with the disorder.

Among common undesirable side effects from drugs are nausea, vomiting, skin rashes, electrolyte imbalance, and changes in the level of consciousness or emotional affect. Side effects may be mild, or they may be severe and life threatening. The less serious ones are often undiagnosed, and in long term drug therapy may persist as troublesome and distressing conditions that are refractory to treatment. Table 23.3 illustrate the commonly occurring signs and symptoms of adverse drug reaction.

Table 23.3. Signs and symptoms of adverse drug reactions

Adverse drug reaction	*Signs and symptoms*
Allergy	Any organ can be affected, including the central nervous system, gastrointestinal system, bone marrow and liver, with signs and symptoms similar to those listed below for these systems
Anaphylaxis	Itching of palms, chin, throat, a sensation of swelling in the throat, apprehension, lacrimation, wheezing, dyspnea, hypotension and cardiovascular collapse
Arthralgia	Joint pain, difficulty in ambulation, impaired manual dexterity
Skin eruption	Erythema, itching rash
Bone marrow suppression Anaemia	Weakness, dyspnea, headaches, syncope, unusual tirdeness or weakness
Leukopenia	Fever, chills, sore throat, drynonproductive cough, malaise, redness or pain in a body area
Thrombocytopenia	Petechiae, ecchymoses, unusual bleeding following minor trauma or from mucous membranes, hemorrhage

(Contd.)

Adverse drug reaction	*Signs and symptoms*
Central nervous system disturbances	
Confusion	Forgetfulness, disorientation, inappropriate verbal responses, anxiety
Excitation	Restlessness, talkativeness, irritability, insomnia, anxiety
Sedation	Sleepiness, lethargy, coma
Gastrointestinal irrigation and/or bleeding	Dysphagia, anorexia, stomatitis (dryness or cracking of lips, swelling and redness of mouth tissues, soreness to burning pain of mouth tissues, mouth odour), nausea, vomiting, abdominal pain, bloody or black tarry stools, diarrhea
Hepatotoxicity	Anorexia, malaise, fatigue, nausea, jaundice, fever, hepatic tenderness, elevated serum glutamic oxaloacetic transaminase, alkaline phosphatase, and/or bilirubin, bile in urine
Nephrotoxicity	Decrease in urination (oliguria to anuria), edema, unusual weight gain, hematuria, albuminuria, and/or crystalluria, progressive azotemia
Ototoxicity	Abnormal ringing or other noises in the ear (tinnitus), increased sensitivity to noise, difficulty in understanding speech, audiograms showing loss of perception, particularly of high tones

Teratogenicity

Some drugs when administered to a pregnant woman in early pregnancy, between the 5th week and 12th week after the first day of the last menstruation, can interfere in organ formation. It can result in various types of congenital developmental abnormalities in the new born. For example, thalidomide, a CNS depressant drug, if used between the 5th week and 7th week of pregnancy, can cause photomelia (shortened or complete absence of limbs) in the new born.

Chemicals or drugs causing this type of adverse drug reactions are called teratogens. They affect the somatic cells of embryo to produce abnormalities. Some effective teratogens, which affect the embryo at a dose level that does not adversely affect the mother, are enlisted in Table 23.4.

Table 23.4. Teratogenic drugs

Teratogens	*Abnormalities in the new born*
1. Phenytoin	Fetal hydantoin syndrome, metal retardation, cleft lip/palate hypoplastic nails and distal phalanges
2. Trimethadione	Fetal trimethadione syndrome, V-shaped eye brows, cardiac anomalies, irregular teeth
3. Diethylistilbosterol	Increased incidence of vaginal adenocarcinoma in female offsprings, in male fetus feminisation but malignancies are not common
4. Coumarin derivatives used as oral anticoagulants	Nasal hypoplasia, skeletal abnormalities, CNS abnormalities
5. Antithyroid drugs	Hypothyroidism, goitre
6. Methotrexate (anticancer drug)	Hypocephalus, cleft plate, abnormal cranial ossification, growth retardation
7. Testosterone and other androgens	Masculinisation of female embryo, i.e. clitoromegaly with/without fusion of labia minora
8. Alcohol	Mild mental retardation, increase in anomalies

24

Chapter

Drugs Uses in Clinical Toxicity

Human poisoning can be classified into two broad divisions :

(i) **Acute poisoning :** It may be self or accidental poisoning. Symptoms appear suddenly soon after the consumption of poison. These symptoms increase in severity, and may cause death if not attended.

(ii) **Chronic poisoning :** Chronic poisoning results from a drug build up over time because more drug has entered the circulatory system through absorption than has left it through metabolism and excretion. Symptoms appear slowly. There is disappearance of symptoms on removal of patient from further exposure.

Classification for Poisons

1. Corrosives

Mineral acid : HCl, H_2SO_4, HNO_3.
Organic acids : Acetic acid, carbolic acid.
Strong alkalies : NaOH, KOH.

2. Irritants

Inorganic

(a) Non-metallic : Phosphorus, chlorine and bromine.
(b) Metallic : Arsenic, mercury and lead.

Inorganic

(a) Vegetable : Castor oil seed, aloes.
(b) Animal : Snakes, insect bites, cantharides.
Mechanical : Diamond durt, powdered glass.

3. Neurotics

Cerebral : Opium, alcohols, dhatura, cannabis.
Spinal : Strychnine.
Cardiac : Aconite, digitalis, tobacco.
Asphyxiants : CO_2, CO, coal gas.

General treatment of poisoning : General treatment consists of :

1. Removal of unabsorbed/absorbed poison.
2. Antidote treatment to nullify the poison.
3. Symptomatic treatment directed towards :
   (i) Drawing out the poison : Vomit, purge, diuresis.
   (ii) Neutralization of poison : Physical, chemical, physio-pharmacological and clinical antidote.
   (iii) Protection of various organs from toxic effects of poison.
   (iv) Symptomatic relief.
   (v) Viatalising the vital centres : Cardiac, vasomotor and respiratory centres.

1. Removal of Unabsorbed Poison

Following methods can be used for removal of unabsorbed poison :

(a) Emetics : If the patient is not vomiting, give 15 g of sodium chloride dissolved in one glass of water. Repeat till vomit is clear. If unsuccessful, then 2 teaspoonful of powdered mustard in glass of water will arouse a vomit. If not, then ipecacuanha powder 1-2 g, finally apomorphine hydrochloride injection can be used to induce vomiting. This injection is contradicated in morphine poisoning. Mechanical irritation of the throat by finger, tongue depressant or spoon evokes instaneous vomiting.

(b) Gastric lavage : This is an established method for the removal of any unabsorbed poison from the stomach. Since the stomach contents pass out in 3-4 hours, a stomach wash proves useless after this time interval. However, in opium poisoning this is not the case. By whatever channel, it may have been administered, it is finally excreted through the stomach. Hence, gastric lavage should be carried out in all cases of opium poisoning.

Solution and substancfes used for gastric lavage include :

(i) Saline solution : 1 teaspoonful of sodium chloride in a tumblerful of warm water.

(ii) Warm water.

(iii) $KMnO_4$ solution (concentrate just to give faint pink colour).

(iv) For alkaline wash : 5% sodium bicarbonate solution.

(v) Sodium thiosulphate and dimercaprol solutions are not used for the treatment in toxic metallic poisoning.

(c) Miscellaneous :

(i) Contact poison (if sprayed on skin, eye or wound) can be removed by washing with plain water.

(ii) If a poison has been injected, then unabsorbed poison can be removed by means of incision and suction.

(iii) Inhaled poison like carbon monoxide or other poisoning can be removed by putting the patient in fresh air or by giving artificial respiration.

(d) Removal of absorbed poison : Elimination of absorbed poison can be enhanced by increasing the urine output by means of diuretic like mannitol, furosemide or by adjusting pH of urine, e.g. acidic drugs are excreted faster in alkaline urine, and alkaline drugs in acidic urine. Dialysis can be done to remove absorbed poison.

2. Antidote Treatment

An antidote is an agent that counteracts a poison. They can be classified on the basis of mechanism of antidote action :

(i) *Physiological antidote* : It counteracts the effects of a poison by producing other effects. Bemegride is used in barbiturate poisoning (opposite action). Caffeine is used in morphine poisoning.

(ii) *Chemical antidote* : It changes the chemical nature of a poison. For example, sodium thiosulphate used in cyanide poisoning converts the toxic cyanide into non-toxic thiocynate which is excreted easily.

$$Na_2S_2O_3 \underset{\text{SCN}^- \text{ oxidase enzyme}}{\overset{\text{Rhodanese enzyme}}{\rightleftharpoons}} SCN^- + Na_2SO_3$$

(iii) *Mechanical antidote* : It prevents the absorption of the poison into the body. Kaolin and charcoal absorb the poison prior to absorption across the intestinal wall. Fats, oils and egg albumin also hinder the absorption of poison.

Absorption can also br prevented by using general antidote which consists of following combination :

MgO	1 part
Tannic acid	2 part
Activated charcoal	2 part

All these substances are suspended in glassful of warm water and given orally. This is universally useful and harmless.

In addition to above antidotes, there are some specific antidotes. These include :

(a) Nalorphine used in morphine poisoning.

(b) Dimercaprol (BAL) used in arsenic and mercury poisoning. Heavy metals like arsenic and mercury have great affinity for SH (Sulfahydryl group) and so they combine with enzymes containing this group and inactivate them. BAL has many SH group, therefore, combines with arsenic and mercury and protects the SH group present in enzymes. The complex formed from dimercaprol and heavy metal is stable and excreted easily.

(c) Ethylene diamine tetraacetic acid (EDTA) : It is given in lead poisoning. It forms stable lead-EDTA complex which is non-toxic, soluble and rapidly excreted.

(d) Penicilliamine (cuprimine) : It is used in copper, lead and mercury poisoning due to its chelating effect. The chelating effect of pencillamine is attributed to presence of –SH group in it.

(e) Desferrioxamine : It is used for treatment of iron poisoning. It accelerates the removal of iron from the body.

3. Symptomatic Treatment

It involves assisted mechanical ventilation, maintenance of blood pressure by vasopressor agent, nutrition by intravenous glucose saline and prevention of secondary infection.

HEAVY METAL POISONING

Metals with densities at least five times that of water are called heavy metals. Many heavy metals are toxic but lead, mercury and cadmium are especially notable. Heavy metal ions react with hydrogen sulphide to form insoluble sulphides. Most enzymes have amino acids with SH groups. Heavy metal ions tie up these groups as they react with H_2S, rendering the enzymes inactive.

1. Arsenic

Symptoms

(a) **Acute poisoning :** It include a burning sensation in mouth and on lips, thirst, difficulty in swallowing, inflammation of gums and mouth, abdominal pain, vomiting and diarrhoea. In severe poisoning, there is cyanosis and weakness. The body temperature falls, the pulse is weak and rapid, loss of consciousness follows and death is due to circulatory failure.

Treatment

1. Removal of patient from source of poison to prevent further exposure.
2. Removal of unabsorbed poison :
   (a) Emesis : It should be done by mechanical means.
   (b) Gastric leavage : Stomach wash with potassium permanganate should be done.
   (c) Magnesium sulphate or castor oil purges the unabsorbed poison.
3. Antidote :
   (a) Dimercaprol injection is given intramuscularly 6 hourly.
   (b) Eggs and albumin should be used for the demulcent action. It prevents further absorption of arsenic by forming a smooth coating on gastric mucosa.
4. Symptomatic treatment :
   (a) Replacement of fluids by I.V. drips.
   (b) Peripheral vasoconstrictor should be injected in cases of peripheral circulatory failure.
   (c) Morphine is used for severe pain.

(B) **Chronic poisoning symptoms :** The main signs of chronic poisoning are skin rashes, loss of hair and finger nails, weakness, loss of weight, sore and inflammed gums and mouth, vomiting, abdominal pain and diarrhoea or constipation. Nervous changes also occur and the breath has characteristic odour of garlic.

Treatment

It includes :

1. Removal of patient from further exposure to poison.

2. Dimercaprol injection helps to improve peripheral neuritics.
3. General nutrition must improve.

2. Lead

(A) Acute Poisoning Symptoms

The symptoms of lead poisoning include loss of appetite and sleep, severe abdominal pain, a feeling of pain in the joints and muscles. The central nervous system and blood forming mechanism are affected in cases of severe poisoning. Lead encephalopathy is characterized by headache, confusion, excitement, hallucinations and convulsions, haematological changes include anaemia, haemolysis and impaired synthesis of haem. The gums frequently exhibit the blue 'lead line'.

Treatment

1. Emetics may be used to expel the unabsorbed poisons.
2. Gastric lavage : Stomach wash is done by sodium or magnesium sulphate followed by pain water.
3. Albumin should be given to prevent further absorption of poison.
4. Chelating agent, e.g. EDTA should be used in injection form. Penicillamine can also be used orally or in the I/V drip form.

(B) Chronic Lead Poisoning

Symptoms : It includes vomiting, abdominal pain, metallic taste and blue line on the gums, chronic constipation. There may be lead palsies (wrist drop, foot drops) and encephatopathy, haematological changes include anemia, basophilia, decrease in platelets, hypertension and nephrities. In females, it also causes menstrual disturbances and abortion.

Treatment

It is done in following steps :

1. The patients is removed from further exposure of lead poison.
2. Sodium or potassium iodide is given orally to facilitate the elimination of lead through kidneys.
3. Calcium gluconate is given intravenously if abdominal pain persists.
4. Chelating agent, i.e. EDTA or dimercaprol, should be used parenterally.
5. In chronic constipation, magnesium sulphate should be used.

3. Mercury

(A) Acute Poisoning

Symptoms : It includes feeling of metallic taste, choking of throat, burning sensation in abdomen associated with diarrhoea. Thromocytopenia and bone marrow depression may occur. There is whiteness of mucus membrane of the mouth with change in voice. Appearance of blood in the vomiting and urine may occur. In severe cases, there is complete renal failure due to necrosis of the tubules.

Treatment

It is done in the following order :

1. A mixture of white albumin of eggs, glucose and sodium bicarbonate in milk is introduced into stomach to convert the mercury into insoluble mercury albuminate. It is followed by a mixture of magnesium carbonate and charcoal in warm water.
2. Dimercaprol injection should be given to form non-toxic complex with absorbed mercury.
3. Penicillamine is also effective antidote against mercury.
4. Symptomatic treatment : It includes the use of morphine (in severe pain), demulcents (in burning sensation), I/V glucose (in peripheral circulatory collapse), cardiac stimulatant (in heart collapse).

(B) Chronic Poisoning

Symptoms : Symptoms include nausea, loss of appetite, abdominal pain, swollen inflammed gums, skin eruption and paralysis of speech muscles.

Treatment

1. Avoid further exposure to poison.
2. Regular antiseptic, e.g. borax powder, is used.
3. A course of dimercaprol or pemicillamine should be given.

INSECTICIDE POISONING

These include organophosphorus compounds and organo-chlorine compounds, e.g. DDT.

Organophosphorous Compounds

These include Malathion, OMPA (Octa methyl pyrophosphosamide) and TEPP (Tetra ethyl pyrophosphate). They are absorbed from all routes.

Symptoms : These depend on the route of entry. Primarily there is headache, nausea, vomiting, tightness of chest, dimunition of vision, etc. These symptoms are followed by sweating pallor, incoordination, confusion, diarrhoea, delirium, paralysis of respiratory muscles, bronchospasm, pulmonary edema, coma and death.

Treatment

1. Stomach wash with potassium permanganate is done.
2. Atropine sulphate injection should be given intramuscularly to control the muscarinic and CNS action of the poison.
3. Cholinesterase reactivators like paralidoxine chloride and pyridine 2-aldox methiodide should be used if atropine sulphate is ineffective.
4. Symptomatic treatment like artificial respiration or tracheostomy may be used, if required.

Organo-chlorine Compounds

Commonly used organo-chlorine compounds as insecticides are DDT, BHC and dieldrin.

Dichloro Diphenyl trichloroethane (DDT)

(A) Acute Poisoning

Symptoms : Symptoms include nausea, vomiting, tremors, convulsions, incoordination, paralysis, pulmonary edema, coma and death.

Treatment

It includes :

1. Gastric lavage.
2. Atropine sulphate IV injection. It relieves most of the symptoms.
3. Phenobarbitone injection may be used to control convulsion.
4. Symptomatic treatment includes artificial respiration, if needed.
5. Avoid fats and oils use.

(B) Chronic Poisoning

It may may occur from inhalation or skin absorption for a long duration.

Symptoms : There is loss of appetite, mental anxiety, insomnia, tremors, convulsion and coma.

Treatment

1. Avoid fats and oils use.
2. Avoid further exposure to poison.
3. Phenobarbitone should be used to control tremors.

NARCOTIC DRUG POISONING

Opium

Symptoms : Poisoning is manifested in three stages :

1. *Stage of excitement* : It is of short duration and may not be manifested if a heavy dose is ingested. It includes restlessness, hellucination, flushing of face, increased heart rate and excitation. The excitement is so much that the patient becomes a maniac.
2. *Stage of stupor* : Its duration varies from few minutes to few hours. In this, depressive action starts appearing. It is noticed by headache, fatigue, giddiness and drowsiness. The eye pupils are contracted, leading to pin point. The face and lips are slightly cyanosed. The pulse and respiration is normal.
3. *Stage of coma* : This is the stage of coma where the persons cannot be aroused. There is no response to deep pain. The muscles are relaxed and reflexes are lost. All secretion are depressed. There is depression of respiration, with feeble and slow pulse rate.

Treatment

1. Stomach wash with $KMnO_4$ solution is done in all the cases to oxidize the contents.
2. It is important to keep the passage clear by an endotracheal tube. Artificial respiration may be used.
3. The body should be kept warm with hot water bags and blankets. Tea/coffee can be given orally, if possible.
4. Once sure that the poisoning is due to opiates, Nalorphine injection should be given intravenously.
5. Bowels should be kept clear by purgatives like magnesium sulphate.
6. Symptomatic treatment : It includes administration of glucose saline intravenously and CNS stimulants, e.g. coramine or nikethamide.

Cannabis Poisoning

Cannabis is grown all over India and it contains active principle tetrahydrocannabiol. It is available in various forms, e.g. bhang, **marijuana,** ganja, charas or hashish.

Symptoms : First the patient is excited and then he has hallucination, laughs, signs, talks loudly, purposeless muscular movements.

After excitement, there are changes in symptoms which include giddiness, loss of coordination of movement, drowsiness, weakness of muscles and dilation of eye pupils. In some cases, the patient is in a state of general anaesthesia.

Treatment

1. Removal of unabsorbed poison by stomach wash.
2. Stimulants may be injected.
3. Artificial respiration and O_2 inhalation.
4. Symptomatic treatment, if and when needed.

Cocaine Poisoning

Cocaine is the active principle of coca plant. It is a stimulant, aphrodisiac, produces a feeling of comfort and increases mental efficiency and muscular power.

Symptoms : Symptoms are manifested in two stages :

(i) Stage of excitement : It includes sense of well being, restlessness, talkativeness and increase of reflexes.

(ii) Stage of necrosis : It is manifested by dryness of throat and mouth, difficulty in swallowing, giddiness, dilation of eye pupil, feeble and slow pulse and convulsions. The patient goes into coma, respiratory failure and the death.

Treatment

Treatment includes following steps :

1. Emetics.
2. Demulcent drinks.
3. Stimulants by parenteral route.
4. Artificial respiration and oxygen inhalation.

BARBITURATES POISONING

Symptoms

There is a coma with respiratory depression, hypotension, oliguria, renal shutdown, hypothermia and pneumonia. Death may occur due to respiratory failure.

Treatment

1. Stomach wash with $KMnO_4$ solution followed with sodium bicarbonate solution.
2. Universal antidote is given.
3. Purgation may be done with magnesium sulphate.
4. Picrotoxin injection is given intravenously. Repeat after 10 minutes but decrease the dose and repeat till refluxes appear.
5. CNS stimulants like bemegride, nikethamide and leptazol can be given intramuscularly.

   Synergistic treatment with bemegride and leptazole incorporated in the drip, in doses of 10 ml of 5% bemegride + 1 ml of 1.5 leptazol *awaken the deeply comatosed patient to* a state of anaesthesia. From this, remarkable recovery follows in a few hours. If not, restart injection.

   These analeptics are toxic, if tremor and twitching are seen, then interrupt the drip. It coma ensure, restart drip.
6. Glucose solution is given by I/V drip as long as unconsciousness continues.
7. Artificial respiration with mixture of 95% oxygen and 5% carbon dioxide may also be used, if necessary.

25

Chapter

Drug Abuse and Drug Dependence

Use of opium, hashish, tobacco, smoking, barbiturates, drinkings, tea and many other new drugs are common in practice for pleasure and satisfaction or to induce sleep or to elevate mood. These drugs have become the requirement for modern people to live a comfortable life. All these drugs are known by different terms, i.e. drug abuse, addiction, drug dependence, etc.

Drug abuse : It is the inappropriate, excessive and persistent use of a drug beyond the medical need.

Drug addiction : It is a state of chronic intoxication produced by the repeated consumption of drug. Its characteristics include :

(i) an overpowering desire or need (compulsion) to continue the drug and to obtain it by any means.

(ii) a tendency to increase the dose.

Drug habituation : It is a condition resulting from the repeated consumption of a drug. Its characteristics include :

(i) a desire (but not a compulsion) to continue the drug for the sense of well being.

(ii) a little or no tendency to increase the dose.

Tolerance

It is a form of drug resistance. It is induced by exposure of the individual to the drug in question. If a drug is taken repeatedly, it is likely to become progressively less effective so that the dose has to be increased to get the same original effect.

Cross Tolerance

The tolerance that develops to some drugs also causes tolerance of drugs of the same pharmacological class. This is the phenomenon of cross tolerance.

Drug dependence : Repeated consumption of certain drugs may cause a habit and dependence which are of two types :

(i) Psychological dependence : A condition in which a drug produces "a feeling of satisfaction and a psychic drive that require continuous administration of the drug to produce pleasure or to avoid discomfort" is called psychic dependence. If the habit forming drug is not available to the habituate, he develops withdrawal symptoms characterized by psychic disturbances like headache, restlessness, emotional upset and/or convulsion and vasomotor collapse.

(ii) Physical dependence : It is a condition in which withdrawal symptoms are manifested by physical disturbances. Physical dependence cannot occur without tolerance. It is an altered or adaptive physiological state of body.

General Treatment

Drug dependence once developed, is difficult to treat. A full cooperation is necessary from the individual. General outlines for treatment are :

(i) Gradual or sudden withdrawal of the drug. Abrupt withdrawal is possible without any harm for drugs not producing physical dependence.

(ii) Specific substitution therapy is based on the advantage of development of cross tolerance. Drugs which produce cross tolerance and less severe side effects may be given, e.g. methadone replaces morphine.

(iii) Psychotherapy and occupational therapy.

(iv) Specific drug therapy, e.g. in case of alcohol poisoning, a drug antabuse is used. Alcohol is metabolized in the following way : Alcohol → Acid → Aldehyde. The end product aldehyde is responsible for the severe condition. Antabuse helps in treatment of alcohol by blocking the metabolism of alcohol to aldehyde.

(v) Correction of nutritional deficiencies.

(vi) Community treatment and rehabilitation.

DRUG DEPENDENCE AND ITS TREATMENT

1. Narcotic Analgesics (Morphine)

Morphine is a main narcotic analgesic drug. It is used in the severe pain due to its CNS depressant properties. Heroin, diacetyl morphine, is more potent than morphine. Due to drug dependence problems, these drugs are only used in compelling situation, e.g. cancer pain.

Withdrawal symptoms of narcotic analgesics : The withdrawal symptoms appears after an abstience period of 6 to 12 hours after the last dose and can be very severe and even fatal. The person develops intense desire for the drug, lethargy and weakness. After 12 hours, yawning, lacrimation, perspiration, rhinorrhoea, tremors and anorexia appear. The peak of the withdrawal symptoms is reached after 48 hours and is characterized by fever, rise in blood pressure, increase in heart rate, dilation of previously constricted pupils and abdominal cramps.

Treatment

(i) Morphine should not be prescribed readily for chronic pain except in cases of compelling situation, e.g. cancer pain.

(ii) Gradual withdrawal of morphine with substitution of another narcotic analgesic to decrease the severity of withdrawal syndrome.

Methadone is the drug of choice in the treatment of dependence of morphine type. Methadone is narcotic analgesic and specific cross tolerance permits the replacement of morphine like drugs of dependence by methadone, e.g. 1 mg of methadone replaces 2 mg of heroin and 4 mg of morphine. Drug (morphine) is completely withdrawn and methadone, at the calculated dose level is administered as soon as symptoms of abstinence syndrome appear. The dose of methadone is itself gradually reduced over a period of week. Cyclazocine, another morphine like analgesic, can also be used in a similar way to methadone.

2. Alcohol

It is the main constituents of all kind of alcoholic beverages.

Withdrawal Symptoms

The habitual consumption of large quantities of alcoholic drinks induces a state of physical dependence. Sudden withdrawal of alcohol results in withdrawal syndrome. Shortly after alcoholic drinking, there is tremor, nausea, vomiting and profuse perspiration. Further drink will arrest the development of his condition but if he continues to abstain, his tremor becomes much worse and hallucination occurs, with fever and convulsions. The syndrome reaches its peak of severity about three days after the last drink. Thereafter, it declines in intensity and individual recovers his normal conditions. There may be associated changes due to nutritional deficiencies such as polyneuritis due to thiamine deficiency. Chronic alcoholic may also suffer from hyperlipidemia, hyperurieamia, hyperurieamia and pancreatities.

Treatment

(i) Tremors of early stage can be prevented with alcohol but long acting depressant drugs, e.g. phenobarbitone and chlordiazepoxide are preferred.

(ii) Nutritional deficiencies and dehydration conditions can be overcome by administration of thiamine/nicotinic acid or other intravenous fluid.

(iii) Drug like disulphiram (antabuse) offers more advantage. Disulphiram is taken orally in doses of about 500 mg daily. It produce no untoward effect but when alcohol is taken, disagreeable symptoms appear like flushing, sweating, nausea, headache, hypotension and respiratory embrassment. Thus the patient is encouraged in his aim to avoid alcohol. Successful treatment depend on his continuing willingness to cooperate by taking disulphiram once a day. Disulphiram inhibits the aldehyde dehydrogenase in the liver, preventing the complete oxidation of alcohol and permitting the accumulation of aldehyde in the blood.

Newer drug, **Calcium carbimide**, also performs the same function as disulphiram.

(iv) Psychotherapy : It can also be useful in alcoholic dependence.

3. Barbiturates

Repeated administration of barbiturates causes drug dependence. The characteristic manifestation of chronic barbiturate toxicity are thick, slurred speech, ataxia, impaired reflexes and hypotoma. Nutrition deficiency, e.g. folate deficiency, rickets in children and ostomalacia in adults, may occur.

Withdrawal Symptom

It appears within 36 hours after the last dose. It includes anxiety, restlessness tremors, abdominal cramps, nausea, vomiting and hypotension. Convulsion with the withdrawal of short acting barbiturates usually develop on the 2nd or 3rd day while they are manifested from 4th to 7th day and are accompanied by cardiovascular collapse. Usually the withdrawal syndrome is mild and clears up by about the 8th day but sometimes may last for many weeks.

Treatment

It is important to prevent the development of withdrawal syndrome because delirium, which is likely to be precipitated by sudden withdrawal, may be difficult to control. In the treatment of barbiturate, short acting drug should be withdrawn and replaced by long acting barbiturate, e.g. pentobarbitone which must be given to prevent withdrawal syndrome. The dose of the substitute is then slowly reduced until about two weeks it has completely withdrawn.

Replacement can also be done by chlordiazepoxide which is also gradually withdrawn.

After complete withdrawal of a depressant drug, it may be necessary to sedate the patient to prevent restlessness.

4. Hallucinogens

The powerful hallucinogens, e.g. mescaline, lysergic acid diethylamide (LSD), depress the central nervous system and cause pschotic reactions. Their effect, other than CNS, are pupil dilation, tachycardia, increased body temperature, pulse rate and respiratory rate.

Treatment

It includes following therapy :

(i) Psychotherapy.
(ii) Antianxiety and sedative drugs can be used.
(iii) Psychotic reaction like schizophrenia may be treated with drug like chloropromazine.

5. Central Nervous System Stimulants

These agents, for example cocaine, amphetamine, stimulate the central nervous system. They produce the psychological dependence. Drug withdrawal produce fatigue, tremor, depression and gastrointestinal disturbance.

Treatment

Toxic manifestations of chronic stimulant abuse, exhibited as psychotic reactions, can be treated with phenothiazines or antipsychotic agents such as haloperidol. If the severe amphetamine withdrawal symptoms occur in the form of depression, they can be treated with tricyclic antidepressants. For psychological treatment, it is advisable to admit in the hospital where patient can be observed in a better way.

26

Chapter

Patient Counselling

Counseling may be defined as "a one-to-one interaction between a pharmacist and a patient and/or caregiver. It is interactive in nature. It should include an assessment of whether or not the information was received as intended and that the patient understands how to use the information to improve the probability of positive therapeutic outcomes.

Patient counseling is a key competency element of the Pharmaceutical Care process. Given the advertising for medication in the media and easy access to information on the Web, it is important for pharmacists to provide appropriate, understandable and relevant information to patients about their medication. The pharmacist is in a highly visible and readily available position to answer patient concerns and enquiries about their medications and alternate treatments they may read about or hear from others.

Outcome of Patient Counseling

The counseling process, properly implemented and consistently maintained, will result in the following benefits/outcomes :

- Improved patient understanding of their medication, resulting in increased compliance
- Reinforcement of advice from primary health care team
- Those patients most in need given more attention
- Improved job satisfaction for pharmacists
- Improved patient loyalty
- Improved pharmacist-prescriber relationships
- Ability to demonstrate quality of service provided when requested by outside agencies

What to Counsel

The following is excerpted from the Standards of Practice document :

(i) A pharmacist must develop, implement and fulfil plans to monitor the patient's progress towards desired therapeutic outcomes

(ii) Routinely and accurately identify the amount and type of education desired/required by patients to maximize their chances of solving or preventing their drug related problem(s).

(iii) Routinely and accurately identify the degree of monitoring required by a patient according to the health risks posed by the patient's medication, drug related problems, or disease.

(iv) Routinely, effectively and, in consideration of the above two statements, appropriately educate patients on the following when dispensing prescription and non-prescription drugs, when patient counseling on discharge medications or when providing recommendations about management of specific drug related problems:

- name and class of the drug (e.g. antibiotic, pain reliever)
- directions for use including education about drug devices
- special storage requirements
- common or important drug-drug or drug -food interactions
- the reason for the drug and the intended therapeutic response and associated time frames (it is recognized that pharmacists do not always have access to the therapeutic indication for the drug).
- common or important side effects and associated time frames
- what the patient should do to monitor his/her therapeutic response or development of side effects
- actions the patient should take if the intended therapeutic response is not obtained or side effects develop
- when appropriate, the actions the pharmacist will undertake to monitor the patient's progress

Who and When to Counsel

The amount and type of information provided to the patient will vary based on the patient's needs, and practice setting. Ideally, the pharmacist counsels patients on all new and refill prescriptions. If the pharmacist cannot counsel to this extent, it should be defined which patient types, or which medications pharmacists will routinely counsel patients. This will vary depending on the pharmacy clientele and may include :

- Patients receiving more than a specified number of medications
- Patients known to have visual, hearing or literacy problems
- Paediatric patients
- Patients on anticoagulants

Pharmacists should counsel on all new prescriptions, including transferred prescriptions.

Counseling on transferred medications may seem to be unnecessary given that the patient has already been taking the medication; however, it provides the pharmacist an opportunity to interact, and establish a relationship with the patient. The pharmacist may determine there are medication related problems or concerns the patient has from this conversation.

Format of Counseling Provided

Counseling should be verbal, and accompanied by written material for the patient to refer to at home. Patients are often stressed and upset from their illness while waiting for their prescription and may not be able to focus on what the pharmacist is discussing with them. Written material reinforces what the pharmacist says and helps the patient recall what was said. If the patient has forgotten or is unsure of what the pharmacist said, the written material may provide the answer, or stimulate the patient to call the pharmacist. This provides the pharmacist an opportunity to reinforce key points about the medication and assess how the patient is doing. The written material may provide basic information only, or be quite detailed. Pictograms, such as those use for illustrating how to administer eye drops, are much easier to understand and should supplement a detailed verbal description.

Counseling Area

The patient should be counseled in a semi-private, or private, area away from other people and distractions, depending on the medication(s). The patient should perceive the counseling area as confidential, secure and conducive to learning. This helps ensure both parties are focused on the discussion, and minimizes interruptions and distractions. It provides an opportunity for patients to ask questions they may be hesitant to ask in public.

Documentation

The counseling session should be documented. This may be as simple as a check list or as detailed as recorded notes in the patients' medication profile. The pharmacist should record (1) that counseling was offered and was accepted and provided or refused and (2) the pharmacist's perceived level of the patient's understanding. As appropriate, the content should be documented (for example, counseling about food–drug interactions). All documentation should be safeguarded to respect patient confidentiality and privacy and to comply with applicable state and federal laws. Any follow-up required should be noted.

The Role of Pharmacist in Patient Counseling

Patients often due to lack of proper information on medication usage, fail to adhere to their medication. This leads to failure of achieving therapeutic goals and decreased quality of life. In developed countries, pharmacists take the responsibility of patient counseling. In India, pharmacists are silent in taking up the counseling responsibility. Major barriers to counseling were identified as doctor dispensing, lack of knowledge, and non legalization of patient counseling.

Since last decade, there is an increasing trend in pharmacy towards the necessity of pharmacist counseling patients on prescription medications. He is a better person due to his knowledge and more ever he also gets sufficient time for interaction. Patient counseling would serve to not only help educate patients about their medications, but would also serve to open communication lines further between the pharmacist and the patient. This would allow the pharmacist to give better health care as he/she would bebetter informed of the patients' overall health, and could further help the patient in leading a healthier life.

In developed countries, specific guidelines regarding how to counsel patients are detailed.

Topics that pharmacists need to address with patients include, but are not limited to the following:

- Name and description of the medication
- Route of administration
- Dose
- Dosage form
- Duration of drug therapy
- Special directions and precautions for preparation of drugs
- Administration and use by the patient
- Common severe side effects/adverse effects

- Interactions and therapeutic contraindications that may be encountered (including their avoidance and the action required if they occur)
- Techniques for self-monitoring drug therapy
- Proper storage
- Refill information
- Appropriate action in case of a missed dose

Example of Patient Counseling

Counseling to diabetic patient

The pharmacist can educate the patients about the proper use of medication, screening for drug interactions, explain monitoring devices, and make recommendations for ancillary products and services. Overall, it is the pharmacist's role to help a diabetic patient in the best possible way to cope with their disease.

Essential components of diabetic counseling include :

- Counseling regarding the disease
- Counseling regarding lifestyle modifications
- Counseling regarding medications
- Counseling regarding acute complications(hypoglycemia, diabetic keto acidosis)
- Counseling regarding chronic complications(diabetic retinopathy, neuropathy, nephropathy)
- Counseling in special populations
- Counseling regarding self Monitoring of Glucose
- Miscellaneous(eye care, oral hygiene, etc)

Counseling of the Diabetic Patient for Prevention of Peridontal Diseases

When counseling patients with diabetes, pharmacists will encounter many opportunities to address any issues they may have regarding diabetes, as well as to reinforce the importance of adhering to the treatment plan to prevent or minimize the complications associated with diabetes. The first line of defense in reducing or preventing the incidence of periodontal disease is the practice of good oral hygiene.

Patients should be educated about other oral health care problems—such as xerostomia, candidiasis, and dental caries—which may be manifested as the result of poorly controlled diabetes as well as improper oral hygiene. Patients always should be reminded that the risk of the development of periodontal disease, as with other complications of diabetes, is linked to glycemic control. Through proper oral hygiene, the incidence of many other health complications may indeed be deterrable.

Counseling Patients About Treating Hypertension

When counseling patients who have hypertension, it is imperative that pharmacists stress the importance of adhering to the treatment plan chosen for the individual by the primary health care provider. The pharmacist also should remind patients that the overall goal of hypertension treatment is to lower blood pressure. In so doing, patients can decrease the incidence of long-term complications, including atherosclerosis, stroke, heart failure, hypertension-related kidney disease, and hypertensive retinopathy.

More than 50% of patients who have been placed on antihypertensive agents discontinue their therapy within 12 months for one or more of the following reasons:

- Adverse effects associated with the medications
- Limited knowledge about the disease and its treatments
- Cost of medications and of access to health care providers

Because the treatment of hypertension involves a multi step plan, pharmacists should make certain that patients clearly understand the required lifestyle modifications as well as the importance of adhering to the instructions regarding taking prescribed pharmacologic agents. Furthermore, for those patients who are started on a pharmacologic therapy regimen, it is crucial that pharmacists ensure that patients thoroughly understand the importance of compliance, including proper administration, dosage, and potential adverse effects associated with the agents prescribed for them.

Initially, some patients may be adequately controlled by the use of a single agent, whereas the majority of patients will require the use of multiple antihypertensive agents. The Seventh Report of the Joint National Committee on Prevention, Detection, Evaluation, and Treatment of High Blood Pressure recommends that the selection of therapy be dependent on the stage of the hypertension, as well as the presence of comorbid conditions, such as heart failure, chronic kidney disease, or diabetes. For patient populations with stage 1 hypertension without compelling indications, thiazide diuretics are typically used. In patients with stage 2 hypertension without compelling indications, the use of a thiazide diuretic in combination with an angiotensin-converting enzyme inhibitor, angiotensin receptor blocker, beta-blocker, or calcium channel blocker is recommended. The committee report also recommends a combination of specific classes of antihypertensive agents for patients with compelling indications.

Counseling Cholesterol Self-Care

In performing patient-specific counseling, pharmacists should recognize current and emerging risk factors and should aim to improve the patient's motivation.

Educate to Improve Motivation

People ignore problems as they do not fully understand. People may hear about cholesterol management but may not understand why HDL and LDL levels are important.

Differentiate Types of Fat

Foods high in fat, cholesterol, and trans fatty acid (TFA) affect cholesterol levels. TFA may be more harmful than saturated fat, but patients are often ignorant of its effects. Pharmacists should counsel patients to read labels carefully.

Review Dietary Guidelines

Fewer than 10% of calories should come from saturated fat, with total fat intake 20% to 35% of all calories. Total cholesterol consumption should be <300 mg/day. TFA should be as low as possible. Patients with unhealthy cholesterol levels must consume <7% of calories from saturated fat and <200 mg/day of cholesterol. Pharmacists may suggest a consumer pocket guide to simplify tracking.

Review Cholesterol-Free Myths

Cholesterol is found only in foods of animal origin. Food labels boasting "cholesterol-free"contents may mislead patients. Many vegetable-origin foods (eg, palm and coconut oil) are high-fat. Also, many fat-free foods contain hydrogenated oils and other forms of TFA.

Stress Cholesterol-Lowering Foods

Several foods decrease cholesterol absorption and reduce LDL. A total of 5 to 10 g of soluble fiber daily from oatmeal, oat bran, beans, cruciferous vegetables (e.g., cabbage, turnips), and fruits decreases LDL by ~5%. Daily walnuts and almonds may reduce LDL by 12%, but they have high calorie contents. Soy at amounts difficult to achieve in Western diets can reduce LDL. Pharmacists may wish to recommend 2 weekly servings of omega-3 fatty-acid-containing foods, such as salmon and tuna.

Encourage Lifestyle Changes

Regular aerobic exercise increases HDL, improves weight and hypertension control, and reduces diabetes risk. Weight loss lowers LDL and reduces metabolic syndrome risk. To track food consumption and exercise levels accurately, pharmacists may recommend a daily log. They also should help patients deal with barriers and encourage patients to seek support from significant others.

Set Realistic Goals

Unrealistic goals lead to failure. The dramatic weight loss by diets usually is followed by prompt weight gain. A 10% weight loss over 6 months is realistic. Sedentary people should begin to exercise 5 or 10 minutes a day, gradually increasing the time to 30 minutes daily.

Get Commitment

People are more likely to achieve goals when they make public commitments and know that others are observing them. Pharmacists should extract commitments by saying, for example, "Tell me how you'll fit in 30 minutes of exercise 3 times a week, " or "How will you limit fast-food lunches to once weekly?"

Think "Brief Intervention"

Counseling from health care practitioners has impact. Studies demonstrate, for instance, that sessions on smoking cessation as short as 3 minutes improve outcomes. Timing is also important. Patients upset with news of 300 mg/dL total cholesterol might be more receptive later.

Putting It All Together

Achieving cholesterol goals frequently requires changing lifelong habits. Toward that goal, encouragement and counseling by a pharmacist can have a lasting impact.

27
Chapter

Bioavailability of Drugs

Bioavailability is a term that indicates measurement of both rate and total amount of drug reaches the general circulation from an administered dosage form. Comparative bioavailability studies determine the relative bioavailability of an active drug in two or more formulations, irrespective of the actual amount absorbed from each formulation.

The concept of bioavailability is developed to observe :

(i) Different formulation of the same drug may produce varying concentration of drug in the blood even though the formulation may meet standard '*in vitro*' testing.

(ii) Difference in bioavailability depending on dosage form and route of administration of the same drug is reported. For example, bioavailability :

Intravenous	100% by definition
Intramuscular	75 to $\leq$ 100%
Subcutaneous	75 to $\leq$ 100%
Oral	5 to $\leq$ 100%
Rectal	30 to $\leq$ 100%
Inhalation	5 to $\leq$ 100%
Transdermal	80 to $\leq$ 100%

(iii) The '*in vitro*' methods of evaluating dosage form provide only indirect evidence of therapeutic utility of drug in gives dosage form. While '*in vivo*' method reflects the safety and efficacy of the dosage form.

(iv) Different manufactures or batches of same dosage form may show variance in bioavailability of drug.

(v) Adjuvants, other excipients and method of formulation affect bioavailability.

In principle, the bioavailability of the drug from oral solution is **more** than solid oral dosage form. Ideally a solid dosage form is compared to both an intravenously administered dosage form and oral liquid dosage form.

If the bioavailability from solid dosage form is lower than oral liquid, then it must be improved by reformulation. Low bioavailability from the oral liquid dosage form indicates that drug is instinctively poorly absorbed or is subjected to rapid metabolism (first pass metabolism) and is not likely to improve the formulation.

Bioequivalence

It indicates that a drug is two-or-more similar dosage forms reaches the general circulation at the same relative rate and same relative extent.

Clinical Equivalence

It occurs when the same drug from two or more dosage forms gives identical result in '*in vitro*' as measured by pharmacological response or by control of symptoms or disease.

Therapeutic Equivalence

It implies that one structurally different drug can cause the same clinical result at the other drug.

Factors Affecting Bioavailability

Following are main factors which affect the bioavailability :

1. Physical properties of drug
2. Nature of the dosage form
3. Physiological factors

1. Physical Properties

(a) Physical state : Liquids are better absorbed than solids, and crystalloids are better absorbed than colloids.

(b) Lipid or water solubility : High lipid solubility of the unionised drug favours its absorption from the G.I. tract.

2. Dosage Form

(a) Effect on disintegration time and dissolution rate : The effect of the physical factor on bioavailability is commonly evaluated by determining (i) the disintegration time which measures the rate of break up of the tablet, or the capsule into drug granules and (ii) the 'dissolution rate' which is the measurement of the drug going into solution. The disintegration time of a tablet is a poor measure of the bioavailability of the contained drug. The dissolution rate is perhaps a better parameter. Dissolution time and disintegration time is affected by other factors, for example :

(i) Particle size : It affectd dissolution rate and so affects the bioavailability, for example in aerosol, optimum performance lies when particle size is between 0.5 to 4 μg. Small particle size is important for absorption of corticosteroids, chloramphenicol and grisefulvin. Thus, the dosage of the active drug can be reduced without lowering efficacy simply by reducing the particle size. On the hand, in case of an anthelimintic such as biphenium hyroxynaphthoate, the particle size should be large enough to reduce in absorption, thus making the treatment more effective and less toxic.

(ii) Crystalline or amorphous form : The stability and solubility of crystalline form are more than amorphous form which affect the bioavailability. For example, procure penicillin and insulin. Amorphous zinc insulin is called semi-lentic while crystalline form is called ultra-lente. Semi-lente is rapidly absorbed and has short duration of action. Ultra-lente is poorly absorbed and has prolonged duration.

(iii) Polymorphic crystal form : The polymorphs (occur in different crystal forms) show different solubilities and rate of dissolution hence different bioavailability, for example steroids, sulfonamides and barbiturates. Cortisone acetate exists in 5 different crystal forms, so there is difference in bioavailabilities.

(b) Effect of formulation : The drugs are absorbed from G.I. tract most rapidly when they are administered in solution. The absorption from suspension is better than capsule and tablets but not better than solution. The availability of a drug for absorption decreases in the given order, i.e. **solution > suspension > capsule > tablets > coated tablets**.

The ingredient of a formulation and various steps involved in the processing of a dosage form strongly effect the bioavailability of the drug. The substances like lactose, starch, calcium phosphate, magnesium stearate and talc, used as diluent, disintegrating agent or lubricant, are inert in nature but may affect the absorption as well as stability of main therapeutic drug. Calcium and magnesium ions reduce the absorption of tetracyclines.

The other factors which may indirectly affect the bioavailability are raw material, type of equipments, methods of manufacture and type of personnel employed.

For example difference in purity or quality of raw material supplied by different manufacturers cause the variance in bioavailability.

If different types of machines are used for the same formulations or there is any difference in adjustment of same machine, it may affect the bioavailability.

There is a well set method for the manufacture of any formulation, slight variations in this, may cause differences in the final product.

Basic characteristics of drug depend on know-how, skill, ability and carefulness of personnel employed. These characteristics in term affect the bioavailability.

3. Physiological Factors

(a) **pH of G.I. tract :** The weak acidic and basic drugs exist in two forms. Ionized form is water soluble and poorly absorbed, the unionized form is lipid soluble and absorbed rapidly. For example, salicylates and barbiturates remain in unionized form in the stomach. In acidic pH of stomach they are rapidly absorbed. Basic drugs, e.g. pethidine, ephedrine, are only absorbed in intestine as these drugs exist in unionized form in alkaline environment. Any disturbance in pH of the G.I. tract affects the absorption which in turn changes the bioavailability.

(b) **G.I. transit time :** The presence of food and its volume, viscosity and tonicity of the gastric contents can affect the drug absorption by modifying the stomach emptying time. Rapid absorption occurs if the drug is given before meals. However, certain irritant drugs like salicylates are purposely administered after food to minimize the gastric irritation. The presence of large quantity of meal or anticholinergic drugs delay in gastric emptying and may result in slow absorption.

(c) **Presence of other agents :** Vitamin C enhances the absorption of iron from G.I. tract. The absorption of fat soluble vitamins is reduced in the presence of liquid paraffin whereas calcium present in the milk reduces the absorption of tetracyclines.

(d) **Metabolism of drug :** Drug metabolism may occur in the liver, e.g. propranolol or in the gut wall, e.g., isoprenaline and so restrict the concentration of parent drug in the general circulation. If the degradation of the drug by the liver is efficient, oral administration results in low bioavailability and sometimes limited pharmacological effects. It is called first pass metabolism.

(e) **Disease states :** Disease that effects the gastric mucosa and function of gastro-intestinal tract, also are capable of altering bioavailability by modifying the absorption rate. Absorption and first pass metabolism, may be affected in some diseases, e.g. malabsorption, thyrotoxicosis, achlorhydria and cirrhosis of the liver.

Methods of Assessing Bioavailability

Bioavailability testing is a means of predicting the clinical efficacy of a drug, the estimation of the bioavailability of a drug in a given dosage form is direct evidence of the efficiency with which a dosage form performs its intended therapeutic function.

The bioavailability of a drug substance formulated into a pharmaceutical product is fundamental to the goals of dosage form design and essential for the clinical efficacy of the medication. Thus, bioavailability testing, which measures the rate and extent of drug absorption, is a way to obtain evidence of the therapeutic utility of a drug product. Bioavailability determinations are performed by drug manufacturers to ensure that a given drug product will get the therapeutic agent to its site of action in an adequate concentration. Bioavailability studies are also carried out to compare the availability of a drug substance from different dosage forms or from the same dosage form produced by different manufacturers.

In vivo methods

One method for assessing the bioavailability of a drug product is through the demonstration of a clinically significant effect. However, such clinical studies are complex, expensive, time consuming and require a sensitive and quantitative measure of the desired response. Further, response is often quite variable, requiring a large test population. Practical considerations, therefore, preclude the use of this method except in initial stages of development while proving the efficacy of a new chemical entity. Quantification of pharmacologic effect is another possible way to assess a drug's bioavailability. This method is based on the assumption that a given intensity of response is associated with a particular drug concentration at the site of action, e.g. variation of miotic response intensity can be directly related to the oral dose of chlorpromazine. However, monitoring of pharmacologic data is often difficult, precision and reproducibility are difficult to establish, and there are only a limited number of pharmacologic effects (e.g. heart rate, body temperature, blood sugar levels) that are applicable to this method. Because of these limitations, alternative methods have been developed to predict the therapeutic potential of a drug. The current method to assess the clinical performance of a drug involves measurement of the drug concentrations in the blood or urine. In such studies a single dose of the drug product is administered to a panel of normal, healthy adult (18- to 35-year old) subjects. Blood and/or urine samples are collected over a period of time following administration and are analyzed for drug content. Based on the blood concentration as a function of time and/or urinary excretion profile, inferences are drawn regarding the rate and extent of absorption of the drug. These studies are relatively easy to conduct and require a limited number of subjects.

Blood Level Studies

Blood level studies are the most common type of human bioavailability studies, and are based on the assumption that there is a direct relationship between the concentration of drug in blood or plasma and the concentration of drug at the site of action. By monitoring the concentration in the blood, it is thus possible to obtain an indirect measure of drug response. Following the administration of a single dose of a medication, blood samples are drawn at specific time intervals and analyzed for drug content. A profile is constructed showing the concentration of drug in blood at the specific times the samples were taken. The key parameters to note are :

(i) **AUC :** The area under the plasma concentration-time curve. The AUC is proportional to the total amount of drug reaching the systemic circulation, and thus characterizes the extent of absorption.

(ii) **C_{max}** : The maximum drug concentration. The maximum concentration of drug in the plasma is a function of both the rate and extent of absorption. $\mathbf{C_{max}}$ will increase with an increase in the dose, as well as with an increase in the absorption rate.

(iii) $\mathbf{T_{max}}$: The time at which the Cmax occurs. The $\mathbf{T_{max}}$ reflects the rate of drug absorption, and decreases as the absorption rate increases.

Bioavailability (the rate and extent of drug absorption) is generally assessed by the determination of these three parameters. Since the AUC is representative of, and proportional to, the total amount of drug absorbed into the circulation, it is used to quantitate the extent of drug absorption.

A variety of pharmacokinetic methods have been suggested for the calculation of absorption rates. For clinical purposes, it is generally sufficient to determine C_{max} and T_{max}. If all other factors are constant, such as the extent of absorption and rate of elimination, then Cmax is proportional to the rate of absorption and Tmax is inversely proportional to the absorption rate. Thus, the faster the absorption of a drug the higher the maximum concentration will be and the less time it will take to reach the maximum concentration.

Urinary Excretion Data

An alternative bioavailability study measures the cumulative amount of uncharged drug excreted in the urine. These studies involve collection of urine samples and the determination of the total quantity of drug excreted in the urine as a function of time. These studies are based on the premise that urinary excretion of the unchanged drug is directly proportional to the plasma concentration of total drug.

Thus, the total quantity of drug excreted in the urine is a reflection of the quantity of drug absorbed from the gastrointestinal tract. Consider the following example : two products, A and B, each containing 100 mg of the same drug are administered orally. A total of 80 mg of drug is recovered in the urine from Product A, but only 40 mg is recovered from Product B. This indicates that twice as much drug was absorbed from Product A as from Product B. (The fact that neither product resulted in excretion of the entire dose might to due to the existence of other routes of elimination, e.g. metabolism). This technique of studying bioavailability is most useful for some drugs that are not extensively metabolized prior to urinary elimination. As a rule, determination of bioavailability using urinary excretion data should be conducted only if at least 20% of a dose is excreted unchanged in the urine after an IV dose. Other conditions which must be met for this method to give valid results include :

(i) the fraction of drug entering the bloodstream and being excreted intact by the kidneys must remain constant.

(ii) collection of the urine has to continue until all the drug has been completely excreted (five times the half-life). Urinary excretion data are primarily useful for assessing extent of drug absorption, although the time course for the cumulative amount of drug excreted in the urine can also be used to estimate the rate of absorption. In practice, these estimates are subject to a high degree of variability, and are less reliable than those obtained from plasma concentration-time profiles.

Thus, urinary excretion of drug is not recommended as a substitute for blood concentration data, rather, these studies should be used in conjunction with blood level data for confirmatory purposes. Single-dose versus multiple-dose-most bioavailability evaluations are made on the basis of single dose administration.

The argument has been made that single doses are not representative of the actual clinical situation, since in most instances, patients require repeated administration of a drug. When a drug is administered repeatedly at fixed intervals, with the dosing frequency less than five half-lives, drug will accumulate in the body and eventually reach a plateau, or a steady-state at steady state, the amount of drug eliminated from the body during one dosing interval is equal to the available dose (rate in = rate out), therefore, the area under the curve during a dosing interval at steady-state is equal to the total area under the curve obtained when a single dose is administered. This AUC can therefore be used to assess the extent of absorption of the drug, as well as its absolute and relative bioavailability. Multiple-dose administration has several advantages over single-dose bioavailability studies, as well as some limitations.

Section-III

Experiments

Experiments

EXPERIMENT 1

Aim : Evaluate the absorbent cotton by chemical test

Procedure

1. **Chemical identification test :** Place the given sample of cotton on a given slide and treat with iodinated zinc chloride solution. The appearance of brownish-violet color indicates the presence of absorbent cotton.

   For preparing iodinated zinc chloride solution, dissolve 20 gm of zinc chloride and 65 gm of potassium iodide in 100 ml of water. Add 0.5 gm of iodine. Shake it for 15 minutes and filter if necessary.

   Absorbed cotton consists of pure cellulose with 6-7% moisture. Cellulose reacts with iodinated zinc chloride solution to form brown violet color.

2. **Fluorescence test :** Place the cotton in a form of fine layer on a glass slide (glass slide should be absolutely dry) and examine under U.V. light. Absorbent cotton shows brownish violet fluorescence.

   Raw cotton is treated with various chemicals to get absorbent cotton. These chemicals may present if not washed. The fluorescence test is performed to check the presence of these chemicals (which are fluorescence in nature).

Observation

1. **Chemical identification test**

Experiment	**Observation**	**Inference**
....	....	....

2. **Fluorescence test**

Experiment	**Observation**	**Inference**
....	....	....

Result

The given sample of cotton was evaluated and found to be.................. cotton.

EXPERIMENT 2

Aim : Evaluate the given sample of surgical dressing by physical test

Introduction

The healing process is a normal biochemical process but use of surgical dressing (bandage, gauge, etc.) speed up the healing process by preventing the unwanted microbial flora in the wounds.

Bandage : It is a babric woven from the samples of absorbent cotton. It is used in the form of strip for wrapping/or binding purposes. It may contain medicament. Bandage should be free from weaving defects, leaf residue, chemicals and other impurities.

Gauge : It is a compact cotton of open texture in multilayer form. It is used in the form of pads to hold the medicament. It should also free from weaving defects, impurities like bandages.

Surgical dressings are evaluated by calculating the % variation in:

(i) length
(ii) width
(iii) thread count
(iv) yarn count
(v) weight per unit area

Procedure

(i) **Variation in length :** It is measured after equilibrating the sample of surgical dressing in a humidity chamber at 65% $\pm$ 20% and 27

$\pm$ 2°C temperature for 24 hours. Unroll the sample of bandage and stretch from one end onwards. Measure the length from one end to other end with meter scale avoiding the wrinkles or creases. Percentage of length is calculated from the formula :

$$A = \% \text{ of length} = \frac{M}{D} \times 100$$

M = measured length of bandage
D = length indicated on the label of bandage
Variation in length (V) = A – 100. The variation in length is indicated by the sign plus (+) or minus (–).

(ii) **Variation in width :** Calculate the variation in width in a similar manner as done in length.

(iii) **Variation in thread count :** Number of threads per unit length controls the aperture of aperture of mesh cloth. This allows the proper ventilation of wounds. Less aperture size will not allow the passage of air for proper ventilation of wounds. The more aperture size (loosely woven bandage) will not exert sufficient pressure on the wound which may lead to swelling.

Thread counting is done in wrap and weft direction. The threads are counted as thread/dm of length or width.

For counting unroll the bandage and stretch on a duck cloth. Put the hollow cardboard block of 5-10 cm over the stretch bandage and count the no. of threads with a fine wire in wrap (lengthwise) and weft (widthwise) and double the number to calculate threads/dm. Calculate the no. of wrap thread count as :

Variation (V) = C – 160
where C = observed wrap thread count
160/decimeter = minimum wrap thread count in ISI unit
Variation (V) = D – 90
where C = observed weft thread count
90/decimeter = minimum weft thread count in ISI unit

(iv) **Variation in yarn count :** Pull out 50 threads of 50 cm from wrap direction and weigh them. Calculate wrap yarn count by :

$$\text{Wrap yarn count (E)} = \frac{W}{25} \times 100$$

where W = weight of 50 threads of 50 cm in wrap direction

Variation in wrap yarn count (V) = 21 – E

where 21 is minimum ISI limit for wrap yarn count

Similarly, calculate the yarn count in weft direction. Pull out 100 threads in weft direction and weigh. Calculate the weft yarn count by :

$$\text{Wrap yarn count (F)} = \frac{W}{L} \times 100$$

where W = weight of 100 threads in weft direction

L = width of bandage in cm

Variation in weft thread count (V) = 25 – F

where 25 is minimum ISI unit for weft thread count.

(v) **Weight per unit area :** Weight accurately a piece of bandage not less than 1 cm^2 from the sample. Determine the weight per unit area as follows :

$$\frac{W}{a \times b} \text{ gm/cm}^2$$

where W = weight in gm of bandage

a × b = length and width in cm respectively

Result

Variation in length

Variation in width

Variation in thread count

Variation in yarn count

EXPERIMENT 3

Aim : Prepare and submit the ampoule of water for injection

Procedure

(i) Distill the tap water in distillation assembly made of neutral glass or stainless steel fitted with a device (baffle) to prevent the entry of pyrogens.

(ii) Reject the first 50 ml of distillate and collect remaining distillate in a suitable container.

(iii) Use this water immediately for preparation of parenteral preparation or fill in a ampoule, sealed (by pulling method) and label it.
(iv) Sterilize the ampoule.
(v) Perform a test for sterility, leakage, pyrogens.

Theory

Water for injection is used as solvent for making parenteral preparation. It has no added substances so it should be used immediately because microbes entered in water may produce pyrogens.

Water for injection is prepared from distillation process. Distillation assembly contain baffle to prevent the entry of pyrogens. First portion of the distillate is rejected as it may contain dissolved impurities.

EXPERIMENT 4

Aim : Prepare and submit sodium chloride injection I.P.

Standard : Sodium chloride injection is a sterile isotonic solution of sodium chloride in water for injection. It contains not less than 0.85% and not more than 0.95% w/v of NaCl. It has pH between 4.5 to 7. There should not be heavy metal more than 3 ppm.

Composition

NaCl	9 gm
Water for injection qs	1000 ml

Procedure

(i) Weigh accurately 9 gm of NaCl and dissolve it in 750 ml of water for injection.
(ii) Filter the solution if necessary.
(iii) Make up the volume to 1000 ml.
(iv) Fill this solution in transfusion bottle under aseptic condition and sealed it.
(v) Sterilize the injection in autoclave (121°C to 20 minutes).
(vi) Perform the clarity test, leakage test, sterility test and pyrogen test.

Theory

Sodium chloride injection is a sterile 0.9% w/v isotomic solution of sodium chloride in water. It do not contain antimicrobial agent.

Storage

Store in a well closed container.

Category

Fluid and electrolyte replenisher

EXPERIMENT 5

Aim : Prepare and submit 5% dextrose solution

Dextrose solution is a sterile solution of anhydrous dextrose or an equivalent quantity of dextrose monohydrate meant for patenteral administration.

Composition

Dextrose	5 gm
Water for injection	100 ml

Procedure

(i) Weigh accurately specified quantity of dextrose and dissolve in sufficient quantity of water for injection.
(ii) Filter the solution if necessary.
(iii) Fill this solution in appropriate container under aseptic condition.
(iv) Sterilize the solution by autoclaving or can also be sterilized by using bacterial filter (sintered glass filter, Grade 5).
(v) Perform the clarity test, test for sterility, etc.

Storage

Store in a cool and dry place.

Category

Nutrient replenisher.

EXPERIMENT 6

Aim : Prepare and submit 10 gm of oral rehydration salt's (ORS) powder

Composition

Sodium chloride	3.5 gm
Potassium chloride	1.5 gm
Sodium citrate	2.9 gm
Glucose	qs to 20 gm

Procedure

(i) Weigh accurately all the ingredients and triturate in a mortar.
(ii) Transfer the contents in a glazed paper bag or wide mouthed bottle.

Theory

Oral rehydration salts is used to compensate electrolyte and water loss during dehydration due to diarrhoea, insufficient water intake. The ORS is a balance mixture of glucose and electrolyte for the prevention and treatment of dehydration.

EXPERIMENT 7

Aim : To prepare and submit 100 ml of dextrose and normal saline solution.

Composition

Dextrose	0.5 gm
NaCl	0.9 gm
Water for injection	98 to 100 ml

Procedure

(i) Weigh the accurate amount of dextrose anhydrous and NaCl.
(ii) Mix by adding sufficient quantity of H_2O for injection in a beaker. Dissolve the contents with the help of glass rod.
(iii) Transfer the content into measuring cylinder and add sufficient quantity of vehicle.
(iv) Filter the content and transfer to the bottle and sterilize it by an autoclave.

Theory

In dextrose normal saline solution, concentration of normal saline solution used is 0.9% because this concentration is isotonic to body fluid. Dextrose is added as source of energy i.e. nutrient. Concentration of dextrose used is 5%. The main advantage of dextrose normal saline is to restrict the volume of fluid intake.

Cautions

Do not use the solution if suspended particles are seen. Do not use if seal of container is broken.

Category

Electrolyte and fluid replenisher.

EXPERIMENT 8

Aim : To prepare 100 ml of Ringer's solution (Compound sodium chloride solution)

Composition

Each 100 ml contains :

NaCl	0.86 gm
KCl	0.03 gm
$CaCl_2$	0.33 gm
Water for injection qs to	100 ml

Procedure

(i) Accurately weigh NaCl and KCl and dissolve in sufficient quantity of H_2O.

(ii) Weight $CaCl_2$ separately and dissolve in small quantity of water.

(iii) Mix and finally make up the volume with water.

(iv) Filter if necessary, transfer the solution after filteration in glass container and sterilize it by moist heat sterilization in an autoclave.

(v) The pH of final product should be between 5-7.5.

Storage

Store in a tightly closed container.

Theory

It is considered superior to normal saline solution because it supplies the required extracellular fluid cations. It is useful for the repair of the deficiency of potassium and calcium ions. The injection is frequently used for treating cardiopulmonary bypass surgery of heat. It is also used to verigate tissue during experiments on animals.

Uses

It is used as irrigation solution to bath and moisten body cavities and for irrigate of wounds.

EXPERIMENT 9

Aim : To prepare and submit 100 ml of Ringer lactate solution.

Composition

Sodium chloride	0.6 gm
Potassium chloride	0.03 gm

Calcium chloride	0.02 gm
Sodium lactate	0.3 gm
Water for injection	100 ml

Procedure

Ringer lactate solution is prepared in two steps :

A. Preparation of sodium lactate solution. It is prepared by dissolving 0.115 gm of NaOH in 20 ml of water for inbjection followed by addition of 0.24 ml of lactic acid. Hydrochloric acid is finally added to neutralise the excess of NaOH.

B. Accuracy weigh the other ingredients and dissolve in aout 70 ml of water for injection. Mix with the solution A and B. Make up the final volume by adding water for injection. Ensure the pH between the 6-7.5. Filter transfer to a suitable container and sterilize in an autoclave.

Theory

It is fluid and an electrolyte replenisher. Its main function is to control the emergency situation i.e. when there is a excessive loss of fluid and electrolyte from the body in evere diarrhoea and dysentry. It maintains the normal electrolyte levels by providing deficient electrolytes which in turn improves the fluid volume. In lactate ringer solution, sodium chloride potassium chloride and calcium chloride provides Na^+, K^+, Ca^{2+} and Cl^- ions respectively.

Storage

Store in single dose container preferably of glass.

Category

Fluid and electrolyte replenisher.

EXPERIMENT 10

Aim : To prepare and submit 50 ml of hemodialysis (acetate 35x)

Composition

Potassium chloride	2.6 gm
Dextrose	70 gm
Sodium acetate	166.6 gm
Sodium chloride	194.5 gm

Purified water 1000 ml
(freshly boiled and cooled)

Explanation

For each 35x hemodialysis required in artificial kidney : dilute 1 L of hemodialysis with 34 L of appropriate type of water (35x).

1 L of diluted solution prepared with purified H_2O contain following ions.

Ions	Concentration
Na^+	130 millimoles
K^+	1 millimoles
HCO_3^-	35 millimoles
Cl^-	96 millimoles
Ca^{2+}	1.5-2 millimoles
Mg^{2+}	0.045-0.75 millimoles
Dextrose	1-2%

Procedure

(i) Weigh all the ingredients accurately and dissolve in sufficient amount of water.
(ii) Make up the volume by purified water.
(iii) Clarify the solution by filteration.
(iv) Pour in suitable container and sterilize by autoclaving.

Theory

Hemodialysis solutions are intended for blood purification. The patients blood is circulated over a membrane of suitable permeability which is in contact with hemodialysis solution.

Label

It should state the strength of solution as percentage or weight by litres for each ingredient.

Storage

Store in a well cllosed container.

Uses

It is used in case of temporary or permanent renal failure to rectify the electrolyte imbalance.

Question Bank

1. Define Hospital Formulary System. Discuss the content of hospital formulary and its organization.
2. What is the importance of Central Sterile Supply Room in a hospital? Discuss the room giving all necessary details along with the qualification of hospital pharmacist to manage it.
3. Discuss the functions and objectives of hospital pharmacy in detail.
4. (a) Name various hospital equipments. Discuss the uses of any two in detail.
   (b) Write a note on 'Drug Information Bulletin'.
5. Discuss the role of pharmacist in prevention and treatment of poisoning. Discuss local and systemic antidotes for poisoning due to heavy metals and narcotics.
6. (a) Discuss any five reasons for increase in number of drug interactions.
   (b) Comment on interaction of Digitalis with calcium preparations.
7. (a) Discuss the role of pharmacist in patient counselling.
   (b) What is the scope of clinical pharmacy in India?
8. Discuss the different types of out-patient services for the Drug-Distribution System in Hospitals.
9. (a) What are the various types of Surgical dressings used in the hospital? Enlist the I.P. standards of absorbent cotton and bandages.
   (b) Briefly discuss the importance of Drug Information Services.

10. (a) Describe the basic plant layout and production planning of a sterile small volume parenterals unit in a hospital.
    (b) Discuss usefulness of Hospital Formulary System.
11. What are various physiological parameters? Discuss their significance with reference to clinical pharmacy.
12. (a) What do you mean by Drug Interaction? Discuss Drug-drug interaction with reference to gastrointestinal agents.
    (b) Give an account on Drug-Food interaction.
13. Define Bioavailability of drugs. Explain various factors affecting the bio-availability of drugs with suitable examples.
14. Write short notes on any four :
    (a) Pharmacist and Patient Counselling
    (b) Use of Computers in hospital pharmacy
    (c) Health delivery system in India
    (d) Drug abuse
    (e) Central sterile services department
    (f) Universal antidotes
    (g) Significance of Adverse Drug Reactions
15. Discuss the following interactions :
    (a) Levodopa and Vitamin B_6
    (b) Digoxin and quinidine
    (c) Albuterol and atenolol
16. (a) Discuss the guidelines for safe and acceptable prepackaging of drugs in hospitals.
    (b) Mention factors affecting selection of equipment for hospital pharmacy. List equipment for non-sterile mixing and filling.
17. (a) How has accreditation improved status of hospitals as health delivery systems in India?
    (b) What are the qualifications and responsibilities of a Chief Pharmacist in a hospital pharmacy.
18. (a) How can a Pharmacist ensure safe, efficient and speedy drug dispensing?
    (b) Write notes on :
        (i) Records of emergency drugs
        (ii) Outpatient drug distribution system
19. (a) Write detailed note on any two :
        (i) Duties of hospital pharmacist in Central Sterile Supply Room
        (ii) Hospital Formulary system
        (iii) Pharmacy Therapeutic Committee : functions

20. (a) Enlist various points that should be covered by the pharmacist in patient counseling of OTC as well as non-OTC drugs.
    (b) Discuss the incompatibility of vitamins with oral contraceptive along with remedy.
21. (a) Discuss scope of Clinical Pharmacy Practice in India.
    (b) Discuss any one method of analysing drug content and their metabolites in blood. How will you correlate therapeutic efficiency of a drug with its concentrations in biological fluids?
22. Comment on the following incompatibilities :
    (a) Antacids with Bisacodyl
    (b) Sulfonylureas with Coumarin anticoagulants
    (c) Mineral oil with Vitamins
    (d) Folic acid with Phenytoin
23. Answer any eight of the following :
    (a) What is Synergism?
    (b) Define Aseptic area.
    (c) What is Settelite Pharmacy Services?
    (d) "Pay counter" Pharmacy Services.
    (e) What if Ward Stock?
    (f) What is CT SCAN and its use?
    (g) What is Glucometer?
    (h) Use of computer in Pharmacy.
    (i) No. of Pharmacists required in a 750 bed Private Mission, Hospital.
    (j) What is Good Hospital Practice (GHP).
24. (a) How do you sterilize the following :
        (i) Eye ointment and solution.
        (ii) Surgical dressings and Sutures.
        (iii) Rubber gloves and Catheters.
        (iv) L.V.P. in glass bottles and cotton wools.
    (b) Pharmacy Therapeutic Committee.
    (c) How do you setup an O.T. Pharmacy Services?
    (d) Draw a flow plan of the non-sterile production area of a 1200 bed General Hospital.
25. Write short notes on any four of the following :
    (a) Testing of raw materials used in hospital pharmacy.
    (b) Drug information Bulletin.
    (c) Emergency pharmacy services.

(d) Drug distribution system in a hospital.
(e) Functions of Hospital Pharmacy.

26. Answer the following :
    (a) Pharmacist in ADR monitoring.
    (b) Pharmacist in patient counselling.
    (c) Setting up of a Drug Information Centre in a District Hospital.
    (d) Write all pharmacopoeial test required for water for injection.
27. Rewrite the following while explaining their interaction :
    (i) Phenobarbitone with Warfarin.
    (ii) Deriphylline with Cigar.
    (iii) Steroids with Insulin.
    (iv) Propoxyphen with Beer.
    (v) Aspirin with Warfarin.
    (vi) Cyclosporin with Ketokonazole.
    (vii) Quinidine with Cemetidine.
    (viii) Vit. D_3 with Phenytoin Na.
    (ix) R-cin 600 with oral contraceptive.
    (x) Warfarin with Phenylbutazone.
28. Answer any four :
    (a) What is drug addiction? Name three drugs which can cause addiction. How it can be treated?
    (b) Write the pathophysiology, manifestation and treatment of pepticulcer and AIDS.
    (c) What is Drug dood interactions?
    (d) Discuss symptoms, complication and treatment of "Alcoholism".
    (e) Role of Pharmacist in monitoring drug therapy.
29. Write short notes on :
    (a) Medication History.
    (b) Gastric Lavage.
    (c) Teratogenicity.
    (d) Clinical significance of Hematological Parameters.
    (e) Drug Induced Diseases.
30. Answer any eight of the following :
    (a) What is "Emergency Drug Trolley"?
    (b) What is "Antagonism"?
    (c) No. of pharmacists required in 1000 beded Govt. Hospital.
    (d) What is Pyrogen and how they are removed?
    (e) What is an ECG?

(f) What is floor stock?
(g) Testing of raw materials.
(h) What do you know about "Bed side pharmacy"?
(i) "Laminar air flow" - its use in Hospital.
(j) What are Health accessories?

31. (a) What are the various systems of drug distribution in Hospital Pharmacy? To you, what should be the "IDEAL" process and why?
(b) The best system of Inventory Control is to do the total computerization of Pharmacy. Justify the statement.

32. Write short notes on any four of the following :
(a) Mobile dispensing unit
(b) Preservatives in injection
(c) Significance of hospital formulary
(d) Centralized and decentralized purchase system
(e) Classification of hospitals

33. Answer any four of the following :
(a) Draw a floor plan of Sterilr production area.
(b) How would you sterilize the following and why?
(i) I.V. fluids in glass bottles.
(ii) I.V. sets and blood sets.
(iii) Glycerine or glycerol.
(iv) Rubber gloves.
(c) Various Pharmacopoeial test for surgical dressing and disposals.
(d) What are various modern dispensing aspects?
(e) Describe the conditions to be fulfilled for all eye preparations.

34. Rewrite the following while explaining their interactions. (any eight)
(a) Smoking and Theophyline.
(b) Metronidazole and alcohol.
(c) Reserpine and digitalis.
(d) Phenobarbitone with phenetoin.
(e) Dulcolax (besocodil) with antacids.
(f) Digitalis with barbiturates.
(g) Aspirin with Beer.
(h) Diuretics with Insulin.
(i) MAO inhibitors and cheese.
(j) Grape juice with erythromycin.

35. Write short notes on any four of the following :
    (i) Patient counselling
    (ii) ADR (genetically determined)
    (iii) Bioavailability
    (iv) Drug induced diseases
    (v) Systemic antidote
36. Answer any four of the following :
    (i) Differentiate the terms "drug abuse" and "drug addiction" and write the treatment of a drug addict.
    (ii) Explain pathophysiology, signs, symptoms and treatment of 'Hepatitis-A'.
    (iii) Steps involved in the treatment of poisoning.
    (iv) Importance of "clinical pharmacy" in india.
    (v) What are the mechanism of drug interactions.
37. (a) Define and classify hospitals. Discuss functions and objectives of a hospital pharmacy.
    (b) Give the layout of a hospital pharmacy.
    (c) Give flowchart of material, men, personnel and facilities requires in a hospital pharmacy.
38. (a) Discuss the role of a pharmacist in patient counselling with special reference to patient compliance. Give example of antibiotic resistance.
    (b) Define Clinical Pharmacy. Give any two of its functions.
    (c) Define 'Systematic Antidotes'. How will you treat heavy metal poisoning?
39. (a) Discuss the guidelines for evaluation of a new/proposed change in a traditional system of drug distribution in hospitals.
    (b) Write a detailed note on 'Unit Dose Dispensing'.
    (c) Discuss Central Sterile Services in a hospital.
40. (a) What does a manufacturing program for hospital pharmacy consist of? Discuss the budgetary control of bulk and sterile manufacturing?
    (b) Give etiology, pathophysiology, manifestations and treatment of Tuberculosis or Diabetes mellitus.
41. (a) Define 'Drug Information Centre' and outline its various activities/functions.
    (b) Define 'Pharmacy and Therapeutics Committee'. Discuss purposes and functions of this Committee.

42. (a) Define 'Hospital Formulary System' and 'Hospital Formulary'.
    (b) What are objectives of 'Hospital Formulary'?
    (c) Discuss the contents of a hospital formulary in detail.
43. Write short notes on (any four) :
    (a) Record of issue and use of narcotics and dangerous drugs.
    (b) OTC counter.
    (c) Procedure and limits of emergency purchase.
    (d) Drug-drug interaction of vitamin D and Phenytoin and Phenobarbitul.
    (e) Interaction of aspirin and antacids.
    (f) Role of pharmacist in prevention of poisoning.
44. (a) What is pharmacy and therapeutic committee? Describe its objectives and functions in drug safety.
    (b) Responsibilities of hospital pharmacists.
45. Describe the process of purchase, procurement and storing of drugs in hospitals.
    Add a note on purchase and inventory control.
46. Write notes on :
    (a) Dispensing of drugs to inpatient.
    (b) Dispensing of controlled drugs.
47. (a) Discuss various types of materials for sterilization.
    (b) Write a note on supply of sterile material in hospitals.
48. Discuss the role of computers and application of computerised services in pharmacy.
49. Describe various functions of pharmaceutical marketing. Write a note on channels of distribution of pharmaceutical products.
50. Define Hospital Pharmacy with its objectives. Give the organizational division of Hospital Pharmacy and also discuss its functions.
51. Discuss about Central Sterile Supply Unit (C.S.S.U.) in detail. Write in brief on materials required for sterilization.
    Describe the sterilization equipment in brief.
52. What are different types of drug distribution system? Give a detailed note on dispensing the drugs to ambulatory patients.
    Discuss the principle of Inventory Control with purchase procedure in brief.
53. Write short notes on any two of the following :
    (a) Role of compensation to Pharmaceutical pre-requisites.
    (b) Budget preparation for Hospital Pharmacy.
    (c) Hospital Formulary.

54. Explain the laws of demand and supply. What is elasticity of demand.
55. List and describe methods of radionuclide production, stating advantages and disadvantages of each method.
56. Define terminology associated with the understanding of radiopharmaceuticals :
    (a) Radionuclide
    (b) Curie
    (c) Bec general
57. What do you understand by Hospital Formulary System? Give an account of its organization composition and functioning.
58. What do you mean by drug interactions? Explain the mechanism of drug interactions, possible problems or effects of the following pairs :
    Digoxin – diuretics
    Lithium – NSAIDS
    Alcohol – Disulfiram
59. Write short notes on the following :
    (a) Surgical dressings
    (b) Drug information bulletin
    (c) Layout of hospital pharmacy
    (d) Significance of various physiological parameters
    (e) Patient counselling and its importance
60. Give the layout, production planning facilities, requirements and economic considerations for manufacture of small volume parenterals.
61. (a) Give the organization, composition and functioning of Pharmacy Therapeutic Committee.
    (b) Write a detailed account of manifestations pathophysiology including salient symptoms of tuberculosis and diabetes.
62. Write notes on (any two) :
    (a) Clinical pharmacy practice in India
    (b) Drug monitoring
    (c) Drug information service
    (d) Surgical instruments and health accessories used in a hospital
63. What are the various drug distribution systems employed in a modern hospital? Highlight the importance of satellite pharmacy services in delivering good health care.
64. Define bioavailability. Discuss the biological factors affecting bioavailability.

Index

Abscess knife, 146
Adhesive plasters, 155
Administration, 15
Administrative equipments, 34
Administrator, 15
Adverse drug interactions, 247
AIDS, 215
Air ambulance concept, 6
Air cleaning, 66
Allis forceps, 142
Amputation knife, 146
Anaesthesia division, 25
Angina pectoris, 208
Antidote treatment, 258
Applications of radionuclides, 163
Aseptic area, 66
Artherosclerosis, 206

Babcock's tissue forceps, 142
Bandages, 154
Barbiturates poisoning, 265
Bard-Parker knife, 145
Bed-side pharmacy, 54
Bioavailability of drugs, 281
Bioequivalence, 282
Blood bank, 21
Blood examination, 217
Bone densitometer, 149
Bone cutting forceps, 145

Cannabis poisoning, 264
Cardiac arrythmia, 208
Catheters, 156
Central supply services, 57
Cerebrospinal fluid examination, 225
Cheatles forceps, 144
Chronic lead poisoning, 261
Clinical divisions, 18
Clinical pharmacy, 175
Clinical services, 18
Clinical toxicity, 257
Computer applications, 134
Complete floor stock system, 47
Control on purchases, 80
Control of quality, 70

Departmental heads, 18
DDT poisoning, 263
Diabetes mellitus, 212
Dietectic division, 23
Dosage form, 262
Drug abuse, 267
Drug dependence, 267
Drug distribution systems, 46
Drug information services, 92
Drug interaction, 226
  β-adrenergic blocker, 237
  analgesic drug, 230
  antidiabetic drug, 233
  calcium channel blocker, 238
  cardiotonic drug, 239
  cardiovascular drug, 234

diuretic drug, 240
drug food, 243
gastrointestinal drug, 241
vitamin, 242
Duodenal ulcer, 214

Emergency drugs, 52
Environmental control evaluation, 68
Epilepsy, 211
Equipment, 34
Examples of patient counseling, 277

Facilities requirements, 32
Factor affecting food and drug interaction,
Surface area, 243
Coated tablets, 244
Dietary metals, 244
Floor stock drugs, 49
Forceps, 143
Features of radiochemical lab, 162
Foley catheter, 157

General manufacturing process,
components, 63
containers and closures, 64
Governing body, 13

Haemostatic forceps, 140
Heavy metal poisoning, 259
Health delivery system, 27
Hepatitis, 204
Hospitals, 3
Hospital classification, 7
Hospital equipments, 149
Hospital formulary system, 81
Hospital manufacturing, 61
Hospital organization, 10
Hospital pharmacists, 37
Hospital pharmacy, 30
Functions, 30
Objectives, 31
Hospital supply, 155
House keeping, 26
Hypertension, 210

Idiosyncrasy, 248
Individual prescription order system, 46
Insecticide poisoning, 262
Intensive care unit,
Intravenous transfusion set, 155

Joint conference committee, 15

Kocher's artery forceps, 141

Liaminar air flow, 60
Lane's artery forceps, 141
Laryngoscopes, 149

Maintenance of records, 123
Management, 13
Medical stores, 102
Medical record division, 24
Medical social service division, 24
Medical staff, 17
Mercury poisoning, 262
Methods for assessing bioavailability, 285
Modern dispensing aspects, 180
Mosquito forceps, 141
Moynihan's forceps, 144
Myocardial infarction, 209

Narcotic drug poisoning, 264
Nebulizers, 149
Needle holder, 147
Non-sterile manufacture, 72
solution, 72
emulsion, 73
suspension, 74
extracts, 74
semisolids, 75
tablets, 76
Nursing division, 22

Organization and operation, 40
OTC medications, 96
Out-patient department, 54
Out-patient pharmacy, 54

Patient compliance, 180
Patient counselling, 273

Pathology services,
Peptic ulcer, 213
Personnel, 66
Pharmacy and Therapeutics committee, 39
Pharmacy division, 25
Physiological parameters, 217
Pricing of prescriptions, 56
Primary wound dressings, 151
Procurement procedure, 105
Production facilities, 65
Production of radiopharmaceuticals, 160
Professional committee, 15
Professional equipments, 34
Protectives, 155
Protection against radiation, 167

Quality control, 77

Radioactive half life, 160
Radiology, 4
Radiopharmaceuticals, 159
Radioisotope thermoelectric generator, 170
Resuscitators, 149
Rheumatoid arthritis, 205
Role of pharmacist, 183, 273
Rutherford Morison's tissue forceps, 142
Ryles tube, 158

Satellite pharmacy, 53
Selection of drugs, 48
Scalpel, 145
Semen examination, 225
Serum creatinine, 221
Serum urea, 220
Surgical instruments, 149
Sources of information, 93
Spencer Well's forceps, 140
Sputum examination, 229
Sterile manufacture, 62
Sterility test, 70
Stomach tube, 158
Stool examination, 221
Surgical cotton, 151
Surgical dressings, 151
Swab holder, 146
Symptomatic treatment, 259
Syringes, 149

Teratogenicity, 254
Terminology of medicine, 187
Tissue forceps, 142
Tongue depressor, 148
Towel clip, 148
Tuberculosis, 203

Ultraviolet radiation, 67
Unit of radioactivity, 160
Urine examination, 222
Unit dose dispensing, 51

Volkmann's spoon, 146